Endometriosis

Endometriosis

Edited by
Emery A. Wilson, M.D.
Professor of Obstetrics and Gynecology
Director, Division of Reproductive Endocrinology and Infertility
Director, Kentucky Center for Reproductive Medicine
University of Kentucky College of Medicine
Lexington, Kentucky

Alan R. Liss, Inc., New York

Address all Inquiries to the Publisher
Alan R. Liss, Inc., 41 East 11th Street, New York, NY 10003

Printed in the United States of America

While the authors, editors, and publisher believe that drug selection and dosage and the specifications and usage of equipment and devices, as set forth in this book, are in accord with current recommendations and practice at the time of publication, they accept no legal responsibility for any errors or omissions, and make no warranty, express or implied, with respect to material contained herein. In view of ongoing research, equipment modifications, changes in governmental regulations and the constant flow of information relating to drug therapy, drug reactions and the use of equipment and devices, the reader is urged to review and evaluate the information provided in the package insert or instructions for each drug, piece of equipment or device for, among other things, any changes in the instructions or indications of dosage or usage and for added warnings and precautions.

Library of Congress Cataloging-in-Publication Data

Endometriosis.

Includes bibliographies and index.
1. Endometriosis. I. Wilson, Emery A.
[DNLM: 1. Endometriosis. WP 390 E56]
RG483.E53E53 1987 618.1′4 87–3948
ISBN 0–8451–4229–1

Dedication

To our patients with endometriosis,
from whom we must continue to learn.

Contents

Contributors

Robert L. Barbieri, Department of Obstetrics and Gynecology, Brigham and Women's Hospital, Harvard Medical School, Boston, MA 02115 **[111]**

Daniel W. Cramer, Department of Obstetrics and Gynecology, Brigham and Women's Hospital, Harvard Medical School, Boston, MA 02115 **[5]**

Robert R. Franklin, Department of Obstetrics and Gynecology, Baylor College of Medicine, Houston, TX 77030 **[173]**

George M. Grunert, Department of Obstetrics and Gynecology, Baylor College of Medicine, Houston, TX 77030 **[173]**

A.F. Haney, Department of Obstetrics and Gynecology, Division of Reproductive Endocrinology and Infertility, Duke University School of Medicine, Durham, NC 27710 **[23]**

Gary D. Hogden, Department of Obstetrics and Gynecology, Jones Institute for Reproductive Medicine, Eastern Virginia Medical School, Norfolk, VA 23507 **[207]**

Mark D. Hornstein, Department of Obstetrics and Gynecology, Brigham and Women's Hospital, Harvard Medical School, Boston, MA 02115 **[111]**

L. Russell Malinak, Department of Obstetrics and Gynecology, Baylor College of Medicine, Houston, TX 77030 **[141]**

Sanford M. Markham, Department of Gynecology and Obstetrics, Division of Reproductive Endocrinology, The Johns Hopkins University School of Medicine, Baltimore, MD 21205 **[185]**

Ken Muse, Department of Obstetrics and Gynecology, Kentucky Center for Reproductive Medicine, University of Kentucky Medical Center, Lexington, KY 40536 **[91]**

John A. Rock, Department of Gynecology and Obstetrics, Division of Reproductive Endocrinology, The Johns Hopkins University School of Medicine, Baltimore, MD 21205 **[185]**

Joseph S. Sanfilippo, Department of Obstetrics and Gynecology, University of Louisville School of Medicine, Louisville, KY 40292 **[161]**

The numbers in brackets are the opening page numbers of the contributors' articles.

Michael W. Vernon, Department of Obstetrics and Gynecology, Kentucky Center for Reproductive Medicine, University of Kentucky Medical Center, Lexington, KY 40536 **[207]**

James M. Wheeler, Department of Obstetrics and Gynecology, Yale University School of Medicine, New Haven, CT **[141]**

Robert A. Wild, Department of Obstetrics and Gynecology, Division of Reproductive Endocrinology, Milton S. Hershey Medical Center, Pennsylvania State University, Hershey, PA 17033 **[53]**

Emery A. Wilson, Department of Obstetrics and Gynecology, University of Kentucky College of Medicine, Lexington, KY 40536 **[xi,1,53,79]**

Preface

As is true with many clinical disorders, our knowledge of endometriosis is based on both factual information, which is inadequate, and clinical experience, which is often anecdotal. If we are to make progress in understanding the pathophysiology and treatment of this disease, we must identify that information which is factual and acknowledge that which is not. Only in the absence of factual information, therefore, can we rely on clinical experience alone.

In most gynecology texts, the subject of endometriosis is presented in a superficial manner. This volume collates what is known about endometriosis and provides comprehensive information not readily available from other sources. It is intended to be a reference source for students of endometriosis and a basis for further studies. To this extent, the contributors have carefully attempted to distinguish factual knowledge, anecdotal experience, and personal opinion. And yet, the contributors have the collective clinical experience to address the many perplexing questions encountered by clinicians dealing with endometriosis and to provide a rational approach to the care of women with this disease. In this respect, this text becomes a valuable resource to clinicians as well.

I am pleased to acknowledge the expertise of the contributors to this text and their willingness to participate in this endeavor. They represent a unique blend of basic knowledge, clinical experience, and zeal for further investigation. I am also indebted to Rosemary Lacey, Darleen Chamberlain, and others at the Kentucky Center for Reproductive Medicine for their help in preparing the manuscript and for their tolerance of the editor's vagaries and temperament.

Emery A. Wilson, M.D.

Endometriosis, pages 1–3

Chapter 1
Endometriosis

Emery A. Wilson, M.D.

Division of Reproductive Endocrinology, Kentucky Center for Reproductive Medicine, University of Kentucky College of Medicine, Lexington, Kentucky 40536

". . . A Riddle Wrapped in a Mystery Inside an Enigma"
Sir Winston Churchill

Although Sir Winston Churchill was not talking about endometriosis in this quotation, the statement aptly describes our present knowledge of the disease. In most respects, endometriosis is an enigmatic disease. Despite many theories, we still do not have a clear understanding of the etiology and pathophysiology of endometriosis (Chapter 3) or its relationship to infertility (Chapter 6). Since the disorder is primarily a human disease and rare in other animal species, the accumulation of factual information has been slow.

Recognition of endometriosis as a disease is a relatively recent event. Although conditions consistent with endometriosis have been reported for over a century, gynecology texts published before 1920 did not mention the disease. Hematomas and "chocolate cysts" of the ovary were known to exist, but they could have had varied etiologies, and they were not known to be associated with endometriosis. The report by Sampson [1] in 1921, describing the histology and etiology of endometriosis and its association with pelvic adhesions, ovarian hormone secretion, and infertility was truly a classic contribution.

Endometriosis is a disease characterized by the presence of tissue histologically identical to endometrium in ectopic locations outside the uterine cavity. Usually, endometriosis is confined to the pelvic cavity, but occasionally it occurs in more distant sites (Chapter 11). In the past, authors distinguished between endometriosis externa and endometriosis interna, also known as adenomyosis. However, adenomyosis is considered a separate pathological and clinical entity with a different etiology, clinical presentation, and treatment. Therefore, except to differentiate the diagnostic features of this disorder from endometriosis, adenomyosis will not be considered further.

We tend to think of endometriosis as a single disease entity, but it actually involves a wide array of clinical presentations (Chapter 4) depending on the extent of the disease (Chapter 5). However, in contrasting the patient with mild endometriosis to the patient with severe disease, it is as if we are dealing with two different disorders. The latter is much more of a mechanical disease with pelvic adhesions and distortion of reproductive anatomy, a surgical disease. The pathophysiology of mild endometriosis, with its local manifestations but systemic reactions, is much more elusive; it is perhaps more conducive to medical treatment if the treatment could only be directed to specific mechanisms. It is, therefore, difficult to discuss the clinical presentation and therapy of endometriosis in general terms. Drs. Malinak and Wheeler (Chapter 8) have designed a clinically useful algorithm for the treatment of endometriosis patients based on their symptoms and the extent of disease.

On the other hand, endometriosis may not be a disease at all, but rather the clinical manifestation of a more basic underlying disorder. Basic biochemical or physiological abnormalities affecting tubal motility or immune mechanisms, for example, could be responsible for the initiation or progression of endometriosis rather than retrograde menstruation per se. In the same converse manner, endometriosis may not be the cause of infertility, but the result of it. The clinical observation that many women have endometriosis but not infertility or other symptoms only underscores our poor understanding of this disease.

Our present bias may extend to the treatment of endometriosis as well. Current medical (Chapter 7) and surgical (Chapter 8) therapies abate the disease temporarily, but symptoms usually recur. Perhaps the principle action of various forms of medical therapy is not by suppression of ovarian function or by direct effect on endometriosis implants, but by "resetting" hypothalamic-pituitary-ovarian relationships, causing ovarian function to improve following therapy. The inconsistent results with therapy again reflect our lack of knowledge of basic mechanisms.

Only in the past 10 years or so has our knowledge of the pathophysiology of endometriosis advanced much beyond Sampson's original description. If we are to learn more about this disease, we must be more critical of the pathophysiological and therapeutic axioms that we now so readily accept. Sometimes our understanding of disease processes must await the technology to explain them. This may well be the case with the immunological aspects of endometriosis, for example, and further technological developments may be necessary for us to fully understand this disease.

Finally, what is the life history of endometriosis? Certainly this disease can develop during adolescence (Chapter 9), but it is usually not recognized until later. Presumably, it progresses in severity with continued hormonal stimulation until menopause, when it regresses. As the disease progresses, it is apt to extend to extrapelvic organs (Chapter 11). But a subtle decline in ovarian function is known to occur years before the climacteric [2], which may influence the progression or recurrence of the disease (Chapter 10), and which may be one reason why more patients with endometriosis do not require definitive surgery.

The first step in learning more about endometriosis is to be aware of the observations of previous investigators, but to be critical of their interpretations. Epidemiological data and identification of risk factors for endometriosis (Chapter 2) can direct our studies. Finally, we must rely on well-designed and well-controlled clinical and basic research, including the use of animal models (Chapter 12), if we are to solve the "riddle" of endometriosis.

REFERENCES

1. Sampson JA: Perforating hemorrhagic (chocolate) cysts of the ovary. Arch Surg 3:245, 1921.
2. Sherman BM, Korenman SG: Hormonal characteristics of the human menstrual cycle throughout reproductive life. J Clin Invest 55:699, 1975.

Endometriosis, pages 5–22

Chapter 2
Epidemiology of Endometriosis

Daniel W. Cramer, M.D., Sc.D.

Department of Obstetrics and Gynecology, Brigham and Women's Hospital, Harvard Medical School, Boston, Massachusetts 02115

INTRODUCTION

The frequency of endometriosis among various populations and how risk for the disease varies by personal risk factors such as family history, delayed childbearing, and other reproductive factors is the subject of considerable speculation. Our notions about these topics have been formed as much by clinical opinion as epidemiologic fact. It is just recently that more formal epidemiologic studies such as population surveys of disease frequency and case control studies have been conducted on endometriosis. Nevertheless, clinical wisdoms often have a way of being rediscovered, which is why the reader will find the classic studies done decades ago cited along with current ones in this chapter on the epidemiology of endometriosis.

THE FREQUENCY OF ENDOMETRIOSIS

Disease frequency may be stated in terms of incidence or prevalence. Incidence of disease is defined as the number of new cases per population per time, whereas disease prevalence is the percentage of the population who have disease at some point in time.

Mortality data are a type of incidence data in which "new cases" are "new deaths" per population per time. Mortality data are a valuable source of information about the frequency of disease. However, endometriosis was listed as a cause of death on only 3 of some 850,000 death certificates filed on females for 1977 [1]. Obviously this figure belies the role of endometriosis as a frequent source of morbidity for women but illustrates that mortality data, a major source of information about epidemiologic patterns, are unavailable for endometriosis.

TABLE I. Prevalence of Endometriosis Among Women Undergoing Gynecologic Operation [2]

Reference	Study population	Prevalence (%)
Long and Strecker, 1939 [3]	Abdominal pelvic operations (n = 1,453), St. Anthony Hospital, Oklahoma City, OK, 1935–1937:	
	(a) all surgeons combined	1.0
	(b) one surgeon alone	4.1
	Histologically confirmed endometriosis only; pelvic sites	
Pumphrey, 1937 [4]	Surgical operations (n = 2,152) on pelvic structures of women, Miami Valley Hospital, Dayton, OH, 6-year period:	
	(a) all surgeons combined	2.2
	(b) one surgeon alone	5.5
	Endometriosis (pelvic and nonpelvic sites) plus adenomyosis (apparent)	
Kistner, 1971 [5]; 1975 [6]	Laparotomies for gynecologic disease, Boston Hospital for Women, as follows:	
	(a) 1950–1965	18.0
	(b) 1950–1972	21.0
Sampsom, 1924 [7]	Abdominal operations for pelvic disease (n = 296), Albany, NY, 1922–1923. Ovarian endometriosis	21.6
Gray, 1949 [8]	Consecutive laparotomies (n = 853). Private practice, Louisville, KY	29.3
Sampsom, 1925 [9]	Abdominal operations for pelvic disease (n = 332) Albany, NY, 1923–1924. Ovarian endometriosis	29.5
Williams, 1975 [10]	Gynecologic operations, author's practice, Mayo Clinic, 1964–1973, as follows:	
	(a) all surgical procedures combined, vaginal and abdominal (n = 5,117)	6.4
	(b) abdominal hysterectomies alone (n = 978)	19.7
Liston et al., 1972 [11]	Royal Infirmary, Edinburgh, Scotland, 1967–1969, as follows:	
	(a) for chronic lower abdominal pain, 134 women	4.5
	(b) for infertility, suspected endometriosis, and other problems (excluding chronic lower abdominal pain), 312 women	8.0
Duignan et al., 1972 [12]	Birmingham, England, 1967–1971, as follows:	
	(a) primary infertility, 520 women	8.7
	(b) secondary infertility, 155 women	4.5
	(c) pelvic pain or dyspareunia, 135 women	8.1
	(d) dysmenorrhea, 27 women	7.4
	(e) pelvic mass, 14 women	None
	(f) amenorrhea and oligomenorrhea, 109 women	0.9

(continued)

TABLE I. Prevalence of Endometriosis Among Women Undergoing Gynecologic Operation [2] (continued)

Reference	Study population	Prevalence (%)
Hasson, 1976 [13]	Chicago, IL, triethnic women, as follows:	
	(a) chronic pelvic pain, 75 women	14.7
	(b) infertility, 66 women	22.7
	(c) other gynecologic problems, 26 women	15.4
Kleppinger, 1974 [14]	Reading Hospital, W. Reading, PA, 1972–1973, as follows:	
	(a) infertility or amenorrhea, 27 women	30.0
	(b) pelvic pain, 28 women	7.1
	(c) pelvic mass, 14 women	7.1
Talbot and Leeton, 1974 [15]	Queen Victoria Hospital, Melbourne, Australia, 85 women, public and private patients, for pelvic pain	21.2
Peterson and Behrman, 1970 [16]	University of Michigan Medical Center, Ann Arbor, MI, 1968–1970, 204 women for previously unexplained infertility	33.3
Bullock et al., 1974 [17]	Wilford Hall USAF Medical Center, San Antonio, TX, 18 teen-aged females selected for diagnostic endoscopy or culdotomy on the basis of dysmenorrhea unresponsive to medical management	50.0
Goldstein et al., 1980 [18]	Children's Hospital Medical Center, Boston, MA, 1974–1979, 140 female adolescents admitted to the gynecologic service for evaluation of chronic pelvic pain after history of 3 prior visits to emergency room, gynecologist, or pediatrician without definitive diagnosis	52.9
Hill, 1932 [19]	Operations for pelvic disease, Touro Infirmary, New Orleans, LA, 1927–1931. Cases identified from medical records search; prevalence calculated as follows:	
	(a) based on all observed cases of endometriosis	10.4
	(b) based on histologically confirmed endometriosis only	9.4

Thus most of the information on the frequency of endometriosis comes from case collections in which the number of women with endometriosis is stated as a percentage of women coming to gynecologic surgery. An excellent review of these reports was compiled by Houston [2]. Portions of her review are summarized in Table I. Two limitations should be apparent regarding these data. First, estimates of the frequency of endometriosis will vary considerably by the nature of the population in the denominator. Secondly, while such data may estimate the prevalence of endometriosis among surgical patients, they do not represent the prevalence of the disease in the general population.

The nature of the surgical population as it varies by performing surgeon, type of surgery, and indication for the procedure clearly influences estimates of the prevalence of endometriosis. In general, the prevalence from personal series reported by surgeons with interest in the disease is higher than that reported by series that include all pelvic surgeons [3–9]. This likely reflects the preferential referral of patients with endometriosis to particular physicians or individual diligence in describing or biopsying suspected endometriotic lesions. Type of surgery may also influence the frequency of diagnosing endometriosis. Operations permitting better visualization of the pelvis are more likely to lead to the diagnosis. Thus series that include vaginal surgery report lower occurrence than those restricted to pelvic laparotomy or laparoscopy [10]. When cases are subdivided by indication for the procedure, sharp differences in prevalence estimates occur. In general, prevalence is highest in women admitted for evaluation or therapy of infertility (particularly primary infertility), followed by women admitted for pelvic pain or pelvic masses [11–16]. A diagnostic group that appears to be at considerable risk are teenagers with intractable dysmenorrhea or pelvic pain. The prevalence of endometriosis in such women who came to operation is reported around 50% [17,18]. The requirement that the endometriosis be histologically proven rather than visually confirmed may also reduce prevalence estimates [19]. Incidentally, some early series on endometriosis included adenomyosis as part of the clinical spectrum, but current use of the term does not include this disorder.

A second limitation of the type of data illustrated in Table I is that it does not reflect the frequency or prevalence of the disease in the general population but rather only in women coming to gynecologic surgery. It may be argued that since the diagnosis of endometriosis requires direct visualization of the pelvis and/or biopsy, the denominator for estimating prevalence should include only women who have had procedures that permit such visualization. Such a requirement, however, is not made for other diseases. We do not require that the incidence of colon cancer be stated only for those who have had barium enemas or colonscopies. The fact that endometriosis may apparently be asymptomatic as indicated by its incidental finding at laparoscopy does not negate this argument. Of public health interest is disease that produces symptoms or causes hospitalization. Thus the commonly stated occurrence of endometriosis around 10% to 15% applies to women coming to pelvic surgery and overstates the frequency of symptomatic endometriosis in the general population.

Probably the best information about the frequency of endometriosis in the general population is contained in a study of discharge diagnoses from acute care, nonfederal hospitals in 1980 [20]. Table II indicates that endometriosis was a "first listed" diagnosis in 0.5% and an "any listed" diagnosis in 0.6% of all hospitalized females. Endometriosis was a "first listed" diagnosis in 5.6% and an "any listed" diagnosis in 7.9% of all females hospitalized with genital disorders other than pregnancy. The average length of stay for women with a "first listed" diagnosis was between 6–7 days.

The national report also allows some estimate of the rate of hospitalization for endometriosis in the general population (Table III). The annual rate of hospitalization for women with "any listed" diagnosis of endometriosis was 27 per 10,000 females of all ages, 45 per 10,000 females age 15–44, and 30 per 10,000 females age 45–65. The disease was virtually absent in girls less than 15 and in women over 65. Women readmitted with endometriosis may

TABLE II. Frequency of Endometriosis as a Discharge Diagnosis in Acute Care Nonfederal Hospitals, United States 1980 [20][a]

Endometriosis as:	Percent of total female discharges by age group					Percent of discharges related to female genital disorders[b] other than pregnancy by age group				
	< 15	15–44	45–64	65+	All Ages	< 15	15–44	45–64	65+	All Ages
First listed diagnosis	—	0.9	0.4	—	0.5	—	7.3	3.1	—	5.6
Any listed diagnosis	—	0.9	0.7	—	0.6	—	9.3	6.9	—	7.9

[a]Based upon a total of 114,000 discharges with endometriosis listed as a first diagnosis and 312,000 discharges with endometriosis as any diagnosis.
[b]Includes ICD 616–629, 179–184, 218–221.

TABLE III. Rates of Hospitalization in 1980 for Endometriosis, U.S. Females [20]

Endometriosis as:	Rate per 10,000 females					
	< 15	15–44	45–64	65+	15–64	All ages
First listed diagnosis	—	18.4	6.7	—	14.9[a]	6.1
Any listed diagnosis	—	45.1[a]	30.5[a]	—	40.6[a]	27.0

[a]Estimated from numbers of cases provided and denominators that can be calculated from data.

be included in these figures, and so these numbers may not represent the true incidence of the disease. Yet these figures are probably as close to disease incidence as any available today. Thus, approximately 4 per 1,000 women age 15 to 64 are hospitalized with endometriosis each year. Such figures are on the same order of magnitude as those admitted with fibroids or prolapse and slightly greater than those admitted with breast cancer.

VARIATION BY AGE, RACE, AND SOCIOECONOMIC STATUS

Just as it is impossible to state a precise figure for the incidence or prevalence of endometriosis, it is possible only to indicate the relative importance of age, race, and socioeconomic status in determining risk for endometriosis. Ideas on the relative importance of these demographic variables best come by examining individual studies that subdivided the study group by these variables rather than by attempting to compare rates from studies in different demographic populations, since such studies are likely to differ in the selection of the surgical population.

Concerning age, Sampson found the peak prevalence to be in women age 30–50, which appears to be in agreement with the national data (Table III) [7]. However, Meigs found the peak occurrence at age 50–59 [21–24]. Although the age ranges studied are too broad to identify the precise age group at peak risk, the studies are sufficient to justify the clinical belief that this disease is confined to the childbearing and immediate postmenopausal years.

Despite an absence of data from the national survey regarding race, there seems to be good agreement that whites are at greater risk for this disease than blacks. Two studies found the prevalence in blacks to be half that in whites [13,25], and other studies reported an even greater differential [26,27] (Table IV). There is also a clinical impression, supported by some data, that the risk of disease among Orientals is as high as or even higher than in whites [13,28].

Meigs emphasized socioeconomic factors in risk for endometriosis, pointing out the higher occurrence of the disease among "private" patients compared to "ward" patients (presumably of lower socioeconomic status). Although race may have confounded this link between socioeconomic status and prevalence of endometriosis, studies comparing "ward" and "private" status among the same racial groups have also shown the positive correlation between socioeconomic status and risk for endometriosis [25,26].

PERSONAL RISK FACTORS

In the previous section, we discussed how risk for endometriosis may vary by demographic variables. How individuals of similar age, race, or socioeco-

TABLE IV. Prevalence of Endometriosis by Race and Socioeconomic Status [2]

Reference	Study population	Prevalence (%)
Meigs, 1941 [21]; 1942 [22]	Consecutive abdominal gynecologic operations, Massachusetts General Hospital, Boston, MA, 1936–1941. Author operated on private patients only. Surgically visualized plus histologically confirmed pelvic endometriosis	
	(a) author's private patients, 400 women	36.0
	(b) ward patients, 400 women	8.0
Meigs, 1953 [23]	Consecutive abdominal gynecologic operations, Massachusetts General Hospital, Boston, MA, 1949–1952. Author operated on private patients only. Surgically visualized plus histologically confirmed pelvic endometriosis	
	(a) author's private patients, 400 women	27.0
	(b) ward patients, 400 women	7.5
Meigs, 1960 [24]	Consecutive abdominal gynecologic operations, Boston, MA, 1955–1958 (private) and 1956–1958 (ward). Author operated on private patients only	
	(a) author's private patients, 400 women	28.8
	(b) ward patients, 400 women	5.0
Hasson, 1976 [13]	Diagnostic laparoscopies performed by author and associates, Chicago, IL. Surgically visualized plus histologically confirmed pelvic endometriosis	
	(a) whites, 136 women	18.4
	(b) blacks, 71 women	9.9
	(c) Orientals, 5 women	40.0
Cavanagh, 1951 [25]	Laparotomies for pelvic disease, Sloane Hospital, New York, 1932–1949. Same surgeons for all patients. Histologically confirmed pelvic endometriosis only	
	(a) private patients, 3,477 women	10.6
	(b) ward whites, 3,099 women	6.2
	(c) ward blacks, 2,060 women	4.2
Scott and Te Linde, 1950 [26]	Gynecologic abdominal operations, Johns Hopkins Hospital, Baltimore, MD, 1933–1947. Surgeons for study population not specified. Surgically visualized plus histologically confirmed endometriosis only	
	(a) private whites, 1,881 women	15.9
	(b) ward whites, 1,861 women	3.2
	(c) blacks, 5,047 women	2.7
Weed, 1955 [27]	Admissions to the gynecologic service, Charity Hospital, New Orleans, LA, 1942–1954. Cases identified by a medical record search that was reportedly more thorough for blacks. Clinically plus surgically diagnosed endometriosis	
	(a) whites, 15,220 women	0.6
	(b) blacks, 28,496 women	0.2

nomic status may differ in their risk for endometriosis is discussed in this section. Frequently information about such personal risk factors come from case reports describing the occurrence of endometriosis in apparently unusual circumstances. Such studies are not formal epidemiologic studies, since they do not contain a control or comparison group and do not allow estimation of the strength or statistical significance of the association. Depending upon the rarity of the circumstance or exposure described, case reports may be useful, however, in suggesting hypotheses about the etiology of endometriosis. We will attempt to distinguish, in the following discussion, associations suggested by case reports versus those established by more formal epidemiologic studies.

Familial/Genetic Factors

Case reports of families with endometriosis date back to the 1940s [29–31]. In a more formal epidemiologic study, Simpson et al. found that 18 (14.6%) of 123 women with endometriosis had a mother and/or sister with the disease, but these same women had only 2 (1.6%) mothers-in-law and/or sisters-in-law with the disease [32]. The women with the "familial" endometrioses appeared to have more severe disease [33]. One may estimate from this study that a family history of endometriosis among a primary relative increases risk for the disease some tenfold. However, no specific Mendelian pattern could be identified, and polygenic/multifactorial inheritance was postulated.

One possible genetic (or at least congenital) mechanism is suggested by case reports of endometriosis in association with genital anomalies, including cervical or vaginal atresia and mullerian fusion defects with obstructed outflow [34–37]. The latter defects appear to have a familial tendency [38] and may occur with a frequency of about 0.1%. Thus the report by Schifrin et al. [37] of 6 with such defects out of 20 adolescents who presented with endometriosis suggests this may be a strong, albeit infrequent, risk factor for the disease, especially in adolescents.

It is unwarranted to conclude from these reports, however, that all anatomic factors that might theoretically impede menstrual outflow increase risk for the disease and therefore should be corrected. Retroversion of the uterus has not been established as a risk factor for the disease and "prophylactic" uterine suspension cannot be recommended. Nor has it been established that routine dilation of the apparently small cervical os is of any benefit in preventing this disease.

Menstrual Factors

While dysmenorrhea is perceived to be a common symptom of endometriosis, the possibility that this and other menstrual characteristics may precede and possibly predispose to endometriosis was recently suggested by Cramer, Wilson, and colleagues [39]. In this study the menstrual characteristics of women with endometriosis manifesting as primary infertility were compared with those of fertile women. Menstrual characteristics were assessed by personal interview (completed prior to the workup that established the diagnosis of endometriosis) and were based upon the usual features of the menstrual cycle when the women were not using oral contraceptives or intrauterine devices.

The average age at menarche (± S.E.M.) for the endometriosis patients (12.4 ± 0.08) was significantly younger than that for the control subjects (12.7 ± 0.01). Table V shows other menstrual characteristics in the endometriosis patients and controls. There was an excess of patients whose periods were "always regular" and conversely a deficiency who were "very irregular" compared with controls. About twice as many women with endometriosis had cycle lengths of 27 days or less compared to controls suggesting that short cycles may increase risk for endometriosis some twofold relative to women with average cycle lengths.

Fewer patients (12.3%) than controls (28.6%) said they had no menstrual pain. Relative to this group, there was a strong trend in risk for endometriosis with increasing menstrual pain. The adjusted risk for endometriosis in women who said they had "mild cramps, seldom needing medication" was 1.7 ($P = .01$). The risk in women who said they had "moderate cramps, usually requiring medication" was 3.4 ($P < .0001$); women who said they had "severe cramps, requiring bedrest" had a risk of 6.7 ($P < .0001$).

Women who reported they had more than a week of menstrual flow also had an increased risk for endometriosis of 2.4 ($P < .002$) compared with women with 1 week or less of menstrual flow. Consistent with a pattern of longer, heavier menstrual flow, more patients (27.6%) than controls (21.8%) required both napkins and tampons for sanitary protection — a finding of borderline statistical significance. Thus there does not appear to be any basis for the concern that exclusive use of tampons for menstrual protection increases risk for the disease. With regard to other hygienic practices, no increased risk was found for women who regularly douched after menses or at other times in their cycles.

The findings of this study lend support to the menstrual reflux theory by demonstrating that the menstrual characteristics of women with endometriosis appear to offer greater opportunity for menstrual contamination, i.e., they had shorter cycle lengths, longer duration of flow, and possibly heavier flow, as suggested by the need for both napkins and tampons for sanitary protection. While such characteristics were assessed before the infertility workup established the diagnosis of endometriosis, they may not have pre-

TABLE V. Menstrual Characteristics in Relation to Risk for Primary Infertility Associated With Endometriosis [39]

Variable	No. (%) of patients (N = 268)	No. (%) of controls (N = 3,794)	Adjusted rr[a]	P*
Regularity				
Always	241 (89.9)	3,305 (87.1)	1.0	—
Generally	20 (7.5)	301 (7.9)	1.0	NS
Very irregular	7 (2.6)	188 (5.0)	0.5	.09
Average cycle length				
Days[b]				
⩽27	55 (21.1)	378 (10.5)	2.1	<.0001
28–34	197 (75.5)	2,979 (82.6)	1.0	—
⩾35	9 (3.4)	249 (6.9)	0.6	.10
Menstrual pain				
None	33 (12.3)	1,084 (28.6)	1.0	—
Mild	69 (25.8)	1,346 (35.5)	1.7	.01
Moderate	78 (29.1)	853 (22.5)	3.4	<.0001
Severe	88 (32.8)	511 (13.5)	6.7	<.0001
Duration of flow, days				
⩽7	251 (93.7)	3,678 (96.9)	1.0	—
⩾8	17 (6.3)	116 (3.1)	2.4	.002
Hygienic practices				
Sanitary protection				
Napkins only	63 (23.5)	916 (24.1)	1.0	—
Tampons only	131 (48.9)	2,051 (54.1)	0.9	NS
Napkins and tampons	74 (27.6)	827 (21.8)	1.4	.10
Douche after menses				
No	222 (82.8)	3,160 (83.3)	1.0	—
Yes	46 (17.2)	634 (16.7)	0.9	NS

*P values of 10% or less are shown. P values greater than 10% are designated not significant.
[a]Adjusted for center, age at interview, difference between age at menarche and index date, education, and religion. Risk for hygienic practices associated with menses are adjusted for these variables as well as pain, irregularity, and cycle length.
[b]Based on 261 patients and 3,606 controls, excluding 7 patients and 188 controls with "very irregular periods."

dated preclinical and undiagnosed endometriosis. Thus, it is possible that some of the menstrual characteristics associated with endometriosis in this study are consequences of the disease rather than precursors to it. In particular, dysmenorrhea is considered a frequent symptom of endometriosis and a likely consequence of the disease. However, an alternate interpretation is suggested by the observation that dysmenorrhea may correlate with elevated uterine contractility [40]. This increased contractility could predispose to greater tubal reflux of menses. By this mechanism, dysmenorrhea could represent another menstrual characteristic indicative of greater opportunity for menstrual contamination of pelvis.

Delayed Childbearing

Meigs popularized the idea that delayed childbearing increased the risk for endometriosis and that early childbearing offered prophylaxis against the disease [23]; this remains a common perception today [41]. The basis for Meig's strong conviction was the difference in the frequency of endometriosis between private and ward patients and the fact that low and high socioeconomic groups differ in their childbearing practices. Obviously high and low socioeconomic groups may differ in many other factors besides childbearing. What is lacking in Meig's data are comparison pregnancy rates or ages at first livebirth for high and low socioeconomic women who did not have endometriosis.

An additional problem in defining this association is that endometriosis may itself cause infertility and thus it may be difficult to distinguish whether the low fertility preceded or followed the endometriosis. Suffice it to say that a formal epidemiologic study has not been performed that can persuasively answer whether and to what extent delayed childbearing is a risk factor for this disease. At the present time, there is little justification to propose that women alter their career goals in some major way because of this possible association.

Exogenous Hormones

In an experimental model, the maintenance of endometrial implants established in castrated monkeys was demonstrated to be dependent on sex steroids [42]. This study supports the theory that estrogen or progesterone is involved in the development or progression of endometriosis. Evidence that this applies in humans is suggested by the virtual absence of disease in girls less than 15 or women over 65 and by indications that menopausal hormone therapy may activate disease [43].

Of greater interest than replacement therapy, however, is the role that oral contraceptives may play in this disease. Since oral contraceptives may lighten endometrial flow, experts have suggested that pills may offer prophylaxis against the development of endometriosis [44]. In an abstract based upon the same menstrual data cited earlier, this protective effect of oral contraceptive use against endometriosis could not be confirmed [45]. Overall about 83% of women with endometriosis had used oral contraceptives prior to their infertility diagnosis, which was in excess of the 71% usage for control subjects. The excess use of pills appeared to be confined to women with moderate or severe dysmenorrhea predating their pill use; and the types of pills used more frequently were high estrogen with more than 50 mcg of estrogen. An obvious problem, then, in studying the association between endometriosis and pill use is that the same menstrual characteristics (such as pain and heavy periods) that may predispose to risk for endometriosis are also common indications for pill use. Additionally, if one proposes that there is a harmful effect of delaying childbirth, then it would be difficult to distinguish this effect from the effects of pill use itself. For this reason it is likely that epidemiologic studies may be of limited value for defining this association. The animal models have not been fully exploited to determine whether the initiation or maintenance of endometriosis is affected by dosage of estrogen or type of progesterone. Such studies may be more important than epidemiologic studies in defining the potential association between pill use and endometriosis.

Another exogeneous hormonal exposure that has been a topic of epidemiologic interest for endometriosis is maternal DES exposure. The ability of DES to cause a variety of gynecologic problems associated with infertility in offspring exposed to the drug has been discussed [46–48]. Changes in the genital tract that might predispose to menstrual reflux have been described [49,50]. However, at the present time it is not clear whether DES exposure increases risk for infertility in general, for endometriosis specifically, or merely represents a bias due to infertile patients recalling this information more readily than patients without such problems.

Endogenous Hormones

Just as there may be some basis for suspecting that exogenous hormones may influence the development of endometriosis, so there is a basis for examining the role of factors that influence endogenous hormones. Again, from the study of menstrual factors, Cramer, Wilson, and colleagues looked at certain constitutional risk factors that may influence endogenous hormone levels [39]. Table VI examines several such factors including weight, height, smoking, and exercise.

Since women who are obese tend to have higher estrogen levels [51,52], it might be predicted that obesity would be a risk factor for endometriosis. However, we found height a better predictor than weight of risk for endometriosis. Almost half of the women with endometriosis were taller than 166 cm, whereas approximatey one-third of the controls were in this height category.

Overall, there were fewer smokers among patients, and one group identified as having a significantly lower risk for endometriosis were smokers who

TABLE VI. Weight, Height, Smoking, and Regular Exercise as Risk Factors for Endometriosis [39]

Variable	No. (%) of patients (N = 268)	No. (%) of controls (N = 3,794)	Adjusted rr[a]	P*
Weight, kg				
⩽56	68 (25.4)	1,143 (30.1)	1.0	—
56–63	121 (45.1)	1,402 (37.0)	1.2	NS
⩾ 64	79 (29.5)	1,249 (32.9)	0.8	NS
Height, cm				
⩽ 160	86 (32.1)	1,339 (35.3)	1.0	—
160–166	62 (23.1)	1,124 (29.6)	0.9	NS
> 166	120 (44.8)	1,331 (35.1)	1.4	.05
Smoking				
Never	151 (56.3)	2,041 (53.8)	1.0	—
Former	42 (15.7)	623 (16.4)	0.9	NS
Current	75 (28.0)	1,130 (29.9)	0.9	NS
Began smoking before age 17 years				
< 1 pack	18 (6.7)	386 (10.2)	0.8	NS
⩾ 1 pack	17 (6.3)	420 (11.1)	0.5	.02
Began smoking at age ⩾ 17 years				
< 1 pack	49 (18.3)	558 (14.7)	1.2	NS
⩾ 1 pack	33 (12.3)	389 (10.3)	1.0	NS
Exercise regularly				
No	203 (75.8)	2,531 (66.7)	1.0	—
Yes	65 (24.2)	1,263 (33.3)	0.6	.001

[a]All risks are adjusted for center, age at interview, difference between age at menarche and index date, education, religion, menstrual pain, and cycle length. Risks for particular exposures were adjusted by the following additional variables: weight by height; height by weight; smoking by weight, height, and exercise; and exercise by weight, height, and smoking.
*P values of 10% or less are shown. P values greater than 10% are designated not significant.

had begun their habit before age 17 years and smoked a pack or more per day. The risk for endometriosis in this group compared with nonsmokers was 0.5 (P = .02). This association is biologically plausible in view of the observation that smoking has been reported to lower endogenous estrogen levels [53].

The final entry in Table VI indicates that women who had exercised regularly also had a signficantly lower risk for endometriosis than women who had not. Thirty-three percent of control subjects said they exercised regularly compared with 24.2% of patients. This translated into a protective effect for regular exercise on risk for endometriosis, rr = 0.6 (P < .001).

Table VII further examines risk for endometriosis by various descriptors of the exercise. The protective effect appeared to be confined to women who had begun their activity at an early age and who exercised more than 2 hours weekly. The types of activity most strongly associated with decreased risk were conditioning exercises, including jogging or calisthenics. Again, exercise is another habit known to affect endogenous estrogen levels. Regular exercise lowers estradiol levels in the follicular and luteal phase. The degree of change appears to be correlated with the intensity of the exercise program and age of the exercisers [54–58]. It is possible that other aspects of lifestyle may influence risk for this disease through their ability to affect endogenous hormone levels. In particular, diet would appear to be a very important area for future investigation through this mechanism.

Other Exposures

Taking the menstrual reflux theory to its logical conclusions, investigators have speculated about other exposure as risk factors for this disease. It has been suggested that intercourse during menses might predispose to antiperistaltic tubal activity and greater reflux. The ability to investigate this exposure in an epidemiologic study would be limited somewhat by the accuracy of the information that subjects might be willing to provide regarding their sexual practices. Theoretically blockage of the tubes by tubal ligation or pelvic

TABLE VII. Risk for Endometriosis by Various Descriptors of Exercise

Variable	No. (%) of patients (N = 268)	No. (%) of controls (N = 3,794)	Adjusted rr[a]	P*
No regular exercise	203 (75.8)	2,531 (66.7)	1.0	—
Age begun, year				
⩽ 15	12 (4.5)	377 (10.0)	0.4	.005
16–25	22 (8.2)	616 (16.2)	0.4	.001
⩾ 26	31 (11.6)	270 (7.1)	1.1	NS
Duration, hr/wk				
⩾ 2	26 (9.7)	373 (9.8)	0.9	NS
3–7	35 (13.1)	713 (18.8)	0.6	.003
> 7	4 (1.5)	177 (4.7)	0.2	.005
Type of exercise				
Walking, hiking	19 (7.1)	283 (7.5)	0.8	NS
Conditioning	25 (9.3)	514 (13.6)	0.5	.005
Seasonal	8 (3.0)	198 (5.2)	0.5	.05
Sports	13 (4.9)	268 (7.1)	0.6	.08

[a]All risks are adjusted for center, age at interview, difference between age at menarche and index date, education, religion, menstrual pain, cycle length, weight, height, and smoking.
*P values of 10% or less are shown. P values greater than 10% are designated not significant.

inflammatory disease should be protective. Sampson reported low occurrence of endometriosis in women after tubal sterilization [54], although a more recent investigation of women requesting reversal of tubal ligation did not support this concept [60].

THE FUTURE ROLE OF EPIDEMIOLOGY IN STUDYING ENDOMETRIOSIS

In general, epidemiology may have several roles in the study, prevention, or treatment of disease. Epidemiology may help identify likely disease mechanisms, may suggest means to prevent the disease, or finally identify populations that should be screened for disease and treated before it reaches more severe stages.

Frankly, I do not see a strong role for epidemiology in defining new leads in the etiology of endometriosis. There have been several good animal models developed regarding the initiation and maintenance of this disease [42, 61–63]. This is not to say that the etiology of endometriosis has been settled. New research may indicate a role for immune mechanisms or prostaglandin metabolism [64,65]. New research notwithstanding, I believe that the animal models have not been fully exploited to examine associations relevant to humans. For example, models regarding the role of exogenous hormones in the maintenance of endometriosis can be used to determine whether oral contraceptive preparations differ in their potency to affect the disease.

I foresee a somewhat greater role for epidemiology in defining strategies for disease prevention. For example, the observation that exercise may offer some degree of protection against this disease suggests a simple preventive measure that would have other beneficial effects on health. The precise mechanism by which smoking may reduce risk for disease needs to be defined to determine whether there are less harmful means of exploiting this mechanism in disease prevention or therapy.

Epidemiologic studies may also help to define populations at high risk for disease. Currently we believe these women to be of higher socioeconomic class, those with early menarche, short cycles, long flow, or with dysmenorrhea. In the future, some noninvasive means for the early detection of endometriosis, perhaps through monoclonal antibodies, may be developed. Women who are identified with early disease may be treated before more serious sequelae of disease develop.

From this author's perspective, the epidemiologic studies that are most urgently needed are those that would define more precisely the incidence and prevalence of this disease. Beyond this it is likely that the epidemiologic studies will be most useful in determining whether factors identified in the animal models are pertinent in humans. Perhaps most productive will be studies that examine the effect of factors that influence endogenous or exogenous hormone levels.

REFERENCES

1. Vital Statistics of the United States, Volume II. Mortality, Part A. National Center for Health Statistics. DHHS Publication 81-1101, 1977.
2. Houston DE: Evidence for the risk of endometriosis by age, race, and socioeconomic status. Epid Reviews 6:167, 1984.
3. Long W, Strecker WE: Endometriosis: review of incidence in 1,453 abdominal pelvic operations at St. Anthony Hospital, 1935–1937, with particular reference to identification and treatment. South Med J 32:489, 1939.
4. Pumphrey RE: Endometriosis: a clinico-pathologic study of forty-eight cases. Ohio State Med J 33:61, 1937.
5. Kistner RW: "Gynecology, Principles and Practice." 2nd ed. Chicago: Year Book Medical Publishers, 1971.
6. Kistner RW: Endometriosis and infertility. In Behrman SJ, Kistner RW (eds): "Progress in Infertility." 2nd ed. Boston: Little, Brown, p. 345, 1975.
7. Sampson JA: Benign and malignant endometrial implants in the peritoneal cavity, and their relation to certain ovarian tumors. Surg Gynecol Obstet 38:287, 1924.
8. Gray LA: The surgical treatment of endometriosis. J Okla State Med Assoc 42:192, 1949.
9. Sampson JA: Endometrial carcinoma of the ovary, arising in endometrial tissue in that organ. Arch Surg 10:1, 1925.
10. Williams TJ: The role of surgery in the management of endometriosis. Mayo Clin Proc 50:198, 1975.
11. Liston WA, Bradford WP, Downie J, et al.: Laparoscopy in a general gynecologic unit. Am J Obstet Gynecol 113:672, 1972.
12. Duignan NM, Jordan JA, Coughlan BM, et al.: One thousand consecutive cases of diagnostic laparoscopy. J Obstet Gynaecol Br Commonw 79:1016, 1972.
13. Hasson HM: Incidence of endometriosis in diagnostic laparoscopy. J Reprod Med 16:135, 1976.
14. Kleppinger RK: One thousand laparoscopies at a community hospital. J Reprod Med 13:13, 1974.
15. Talbot HM, Leeton J: The role of laparoscopy in 1,400 patients. Med J Aust 1:36, 1974.
16. Peterson EP, Behrman SJ: Laparoscopy of the infertile patient. Obstet Gynecol 36:363, 1970.
17. Bullock JL, Massey FM, Gambrell RD: Symptomatic endometriosis in teen-agers: a reappraisal. Obstet Gynecol 43:896, 1974.
18. Goldstein DP, deCholnoky C, Emans SJ, et al.: Laparoscopy on the diagnosis and management of pelvic pain in adolescents. J Reprod Med 24:251, 1980.
19. Hill LL Jr: Aberrant endometrium. Am J Surg 18:303, 1932.
20. National Center for Health Statistics, McCarthy E: Inpatient utilization of short-stay hospitals by diagnosis: United States, 1980. Hyattsville, MD: National Center for Health Statistics, 1982. (Vital and health statistics, series 13: Data from the National Health Survey, no. 74) (DHHS publication no. (PHS) 83-1735).

21. Meigs JV: Endometriosis: its significance. Ann Surg 114:866, 1941.
22. Meigs JV: Gynecology: endometriosis. N Engl J Med 226:147, 1942.
23. Meigs JV: Endometriosis. Etiologic role of marriage, age and parity: conservative treatment. Obstet Gynecol 2:46, 1953.
24. Meigs JV: An interest in endometriosis and its consequences. Am J Obstet Gynecol 79:625, 1960.
25. Cavanagh WV: Fertility in the etiology of endometriosis. Am J Obstet Gynecol 61:539, 1951.
26. Scott RB, Te Linde, RW: External endometriosis: the scourge of the private patient. Ann Surg 131:697, 1950.
27. Weed JC: Endometriosis in the Negro. Ann Surg 141:615, 1955.
28. Miyazawa K: Incidence of endometriosis among Japanese women. Obstet Gynecol 48:407, 1976.
29. Goodall JR: "Endometriosis." Philadelphia: Lippincott, 1943.
30. Frey GH: The familial occurrence of endometriosis. Am J Obstet Gynecol 73:418, 1957.
31. Ranney B: Endometriosis IV. Hereditary tendency. Obstet Gynecol 37:734, 1971.
32. Simpson JL, Elias S, Malinak LR, Buttram VC: Heritable aspects of endometriosis. I. Genetic studies. Am J Obstet Gynecol 137:327, 1980.
33. Malinak LR, Buttram VC, Elias S, Simpson JL: Heritable aspects of endometriosis. II. Clinical characteristics of familial endometriosis. Am J Obstet Gynecol 137:332, 1980.
34. Hanton EM, Malkasian GD, Docherty MD, Pratt JH: Endometriosis associated with complete or partial obstruction of menstrual egress. Obstet Gynecol 28:626, 1966.
35. Fallas RE: Endometriosis. Demonstration for the Sampson theory by a human anomaly. Am J Obstet Gynecol 72:556, 1956.
36. Carpenter RJ, Jameson WJ: Uterus bicornis with rudimentary horn. Am J Obstet Gynecol 116:973, 1973.
37. Schifrin BS, Erez S, Moore JG: Teen-age endometriosis. Am J Obstet Gynecol 116:973, 1973.
38. Simpson JL: "Disorders of Sexual Differentiation. Etiology and Clinical Definition." New York: Academic Press, 1976.
39. Cramer DW, Wilson E, Stillman RJ, Berger MJ, Belisle S, Schiff I, albrecht B, Gibson M, Stadel BV, Schoenbaun SC: The relation of endometriosis to menstrual characteristics, smoking, and exercise. JAMA 255:1904, 1985.
40. Schulman H, Duvivier R, Blattner MS: The uterine contractility index: a research and diagnostic tool in dysmenorrhea. Am J Obstet 145:1049, 1983.
41. Feldman C: Postponing pregnancy may encourage endometriosis (interview with VC Buttram, Jr). Houston Chronicle, December 4, 1980.
42. DiZerega GS, Barber DL, Hodgen GD: Endometriosis: Role of ovarian steroids in initiation, maintenance, and suppression. Fertil Steril 33:649, 1980.
43. Ranney B: Endometriosis: pathogenesis, symptoms, and findings. Clin Obstet Gynecol 23:865, 1980.
44. Novak ER, Woodruff JD: "Gynecologic and Obstetric Pathology, with Clinical and Endocrine Relations." 8th ed. Philadelphia: WB Saunders, 1979.
45. Cramer DW, Wilson E, Stillman R, et al.: The association of endometriosis with oral contraceptive use. Abstract 328. Am Fertil Soc, Toronto, 1986.
46. Berger MJ, Goldstein DP: Impaired reproductive performance in DES exposed women. Obstet Gynecol 55:25, 1980.
47. Stillman RA: In utero exposure to diethylstilbestrol. Adverse effects on the reproductive performance in male and female offspring. Am J Obstet Gynecol 142:905, 1982.

48. Haney AF: Causes of infertility in sixteen women exposed to diethylstilbestrol in utero. Fertil Steril (Abstract) 35:258, 1981.
49. Stillman RJ, Miller LC: Diethylstilbestrol exposure in utero and endometriosis in infertile females. Fertil Steril 41:369, 1984.
50. Kaufman RH, Adam F, Binder GL, et al.: Upper genital tract changes and pregnancy outcome in offspring exposed to diethylstilbestrol. Am J Obstet Gynecol 137:299, 1980.
51. Bates GW, Whitworth NS: Effect of body weight reduction on plasma androgens in obese infertile women. Fertil Steril 38:406, 1982.
52. Siiteri PH, Schwartz PE, MacDonald PC: Estrogen receptors and the estrone hypothesis in relationship to endometrial and breast cancer. Gynecol Oncol 2:228, 1974.
53. MacMahon B, Trichopoulous D, Cole P, et al.: Cigarette smoking and urinary estrogens. N Engl J Med 307:1062, 1982.
54. Dale E, Gerlach DH, Wilhite AL: Menstrual dysfunction in distance runners. Am J Obstet Gynecol 54:47, 1979.
55. Bonen A, Belcastro AN, Ling WY, et al.: Profiles of selected hormones during menstrual cycles of teenage athletes. Am Physiol Soc 50:545, 1981.
56. Baker ER, Mathur RS, Kirk RF, et al.: Female runners and secondary amenorrhea: correlation with age, parity, mileage and plasma hormonal and sex-hormone-binding globulin concentrations. Fertil Steril 36:183, 1981.
57. Boyden TW, Pamenter RW, Stanforth P, et al.: Sex steroids and endurance running in women. Fertil Steril 39:629, 1983.
58. Schwartz B, Cumming DC, Riordan E, et al.: Exercise-associated amenorrhea: a distinct entity? Am J Obstet Gynecol 141:662, 1981.
59. Sampson JA: The development of the implantation theory for the origin of peritoneal endometriosis. Am J Obstet Gynecol 40:549, 1940.
60. Dodge ST, Pumphrey RS, Miyazawa K: Peritoneal endometriosis in women requesting reversal of sterilization. Fertil Steril 45:774, 1986.
61. Telinde RW, Scott RE: Experimental endometriosis. Am J Obstet Gynecol 60:1147, 1950.
62. Schenken RS, Asch RH, Williams RF, Hodgen GD: Etiology of infertility in monkeys with endometriosis: luteinized unruptured follicles, luteal phase defects, pelvic adhesions, spontaneous abortions. Fertil Steril 41:122, 1984.
63. Vernon MW, Wilson EA: Studies on the surgical induction of endometriosis in the rat. Fertil Steril 44:684, 1985.
64. Dmowski WP, Steele RW, Baker GF: Deficient cellular immunity in endometriosis. Am J Obstet Gynecol 141:377, 1981.
65. Drake TS, O'Brien WF, Ramwell PW, Metz SA: Peritoneal fluid thromboxane B_2 and 6-keto prostaglandin $F_{1\alpha}$ in endometriosis. Am J Obstet Gynecol 140:401, 1981.

Endometriosis, pages 23–51

Chapter 3
Endometriosis: Pathogenesis and Pathophysiology

A. F. Haney, M.D.

Department of Obstetrics and Gynecology, Duke University Medical Center, Durham, North Carolina 27710

INTRODUCTION

The large volume of scientific articles and reviews on endometriosis is evidence of the long and continuing interest in the subject by gynecologists and pathologists. It is of obvious import to the gynecologist, as it is an extremely common gynecologic disease, responsible for a significant portion of gynecologic operations. Almost as important as the numbers, young women with endometriosis are frequently faced with difficult decisions regarding their future reproduction. As one of its main symptoms is infertility, there has been a renewed interest in this disease, paralleling the rising utilization of infertility services in the United States [1].

Most clinicians' concepts of endometriosis still reflect the views of the descriptive morphologists at the turn of the century. The finding of cyclic endometrium at ectopic locations provided the pathologist with the basic concept of hormonal control of the endometrium. This descriptive approach has continued to the present with peritoneal endoscopy allowing direct visualization of the pelvic cavity on an outpatient basis. Unfortunately, progress in understanding the pathophysiology of this disease, its natural history, and the mechanism by which it lowers fecundity has been slow in coming. This is of critical importance, as the most common complaint of women with endometriosis today is infertility, and the current therapeutic options have little demonstrated efficacy [2]. The recent development of a subspeciality of obstetrics and gynecology focusing on reproduction should help to infuse new energy into this effort. This chapter attempts to characterize what is known about the development of the disease and its pathology.

DEFINITION

The term endometriosis is defined pathologically by the presence of tissue outside the uterus that is histologically identical to endometrium. Previously, ectopic endometrium had been separated into that which occurred within the myometrium or beyond the uterine serosa. These were termed direct and indirect endometriosis as well as endometriosis interna and endometriosis externa. Clinical observations suggest that endometrial tissue within the myometrium is a separate pathologic entity with a different patient population, etiology, and clinical course [3]. Accordingly, endometrial tissue within the myometrium, i.e., adenomyosis, will not be considered further.

Ectopically-implanted endometrium rarely has the identical microscopic appearance or architecture of normal endometrium in situ. Pathologists have required the presence of glands, stroma, and evidence of menstrual cyclicity (tissue hemorrhage or hemosiderin-laden macrophages) to categorically make the diagnosis. These have gradually been adopted as a rigid criteria for making the diagnosis despite not having significant validation. This seems curious, as menstrual shedding of endometrium occurs as clumps and isolated cells rather than intact fragments of endometrium [3]. Accordingly, it would be anticipated that the implants would be composed of isolated scattered glandular and stroma components rather than exact copies of intrauterine endometrium. Furthermore, the viability, transplantability, hormonal responsiveness, longevity, and functional capability remain unanswered questions. It should be noted that endometriosis is very accurately diagnosed by visual inspection of the pelvis, and histologic confirmation is not mandatory for clinical decision making. For purposes of this review, endometriosis will be defined by the presence of endometrial glands, stroma, or both, with or without evidence of menstrual cyclicity (hemosiderin-laden macrophages), outside the uterine corpus.

EPIDEMIOLOGY

No definitive epidemiologic studies of endometriosis are available. It is clear, however, that it is predominately a disease of reproductive-age women, with the implication that ovarian function is necessary for the development and maintenance of ectopic implants. Likewise, the true incidence of the disease in the American population is biased by the awareness of the disorder and the diagnostic methods available. Prior to the advent of laparoscopy, only cases of endometriosis with severe enough symptoms or palpable findings warranting laparotomy were identified, and the patients were typically in their late thirties and early forties [4,5]. With the use of outpatient endoscopy, the typical age at diagnosis has dropped significantly and is currently in the range of 25 to 29 years of age [6,7]. Significantly, a recent report suggests that the mean age at the onset of symptoms is 20, substantially earlier than the mean age of diagnosis [6]. A further decline in the average age of diagnosis is to be expected with an increased appreciation of the frequency of this disorder in women with infertility and the availability of laparoscopy.

As a functioning ovary is required for development of a normal endometrium, it is not surprising that it is not reported in the prepubertal years. Endometriosis, however, is not rare under age 20, but a separation should be made between disease occurring in the first few years after menarche and that later in the second decade of life [8]. Early disease contains a disproportionately large number of cases associated with Müllerian anomalies, specifically uterine outflow obstruction [8–11]. It is not unusual to encounter the disease in the late teenage years in the presence of a normal genital tract [12,13] (See Chapter 9).

Endometriosis has not been reported prior to puberty presumably because of the requirement for reproductive hormones. After establishment of ectopic implants during the reproductive years, however, it can persist after the climacteric. Endometriosis has been reported in 2% to 4% of women undergoing laparotomies in the postmenopausal years [14–15]. Two factors are likely to enter into the maintenance of the disease after menopause, the use of estrogen replacement therapy and high endogenous circulating estrogen levels due to obesity. With the increasing use of estrogen replacement therapy, more cases of endometriosis in the postmenopausal age group should be forthcoming.

As stated in Chapter 2, the actual incidence of endometriosis is difficult to establish. Reports vary from 1% to 50% of the patients studied, based on a variety of selection criteria including disease severity, occurrence of particular symptoms, and referral patterns [17–19]. The "true" incidence in the general population of reproductive-aged women is best estimated by Strathy et al., who noted endometriosis in 2% of asymptomatic women undergoing tubal ligations [12]. Obviously some bias is introduced by the use of asymptomatic multiparous women, but it does support a true incidence of 5% or less in the general population.

Endometriosis was originally believed to have a strong racial preponderance, with Meigs finding endometriosis in 28% of white women and in only 5.8% black women undergoing laparotomies[20]. These results, however, were not controlled for confounding variables such as cultural differences regarding childbearing patterns, availability of health care, attitudes toward menses and pain, and access to contraception. After controlling for these confounding variables of culture and socioeconomic status rather than race alone, the apparently higher rate of endometriosis in white women disappears [21–24]. Similarly, the suggested links of endometriosis to occupation, education, and geography are probably artifacts of study design.

A long suspected genetic influence on the occurrence of endometriosis was supported by Ranney, in 1971, who identified what appeared to be a hereditary pattern of the disease [25]. Additional studies have subsequently demonstrated what appears to be a polygenetic or multifactorial mode of inheritance with endometriosis occurring in approximately 7% of first-degree female relatives of affected women [26,27] and 2% of second-degree female relatives [28]. Furthermore, the genetic link appears to be through a maternal inheritance pattern [28]. No clearer definition of this genetic influence has emerged, and, specifically, there is no obvious relationship to HLA-cell surface antigens [29].

PATHOGENESIS

The recognition of endometriosis as a unique disease process is easy to understand in light of its invasive but nonneoplastic growth pattern, the presence of histologically normal endometrium at ectopic sites, and evidence of hormonal responsiveness with menstrual cyclicity. Von Rokitansky provided the first detailed description of endometriosis in 1860 [30], and many theories of pathogenesis have been forwarded since that time. As the descriptive morphologists of that era were not experimentalists, it is not surprising that the first theory regarding the development of the disease was that of celomic metaplasia, put forward by Robert Meyer, a major figure in gynecologic pathology at that time. This theory explained the development of the disease by a process of continued tissue differentiation of the original celomic membrane by metaplasia. It was felt that this tissue differentiation could occur in adults in selective tissues despite a lack of experimental evidence supporting this concept. This view of the pathogenesis of endometriosis had wide support in the early part of the century and this continues to be popular today. There are, however, several problems with this concept, and they include:

1) Endometriosis is confined to women. While there are several case reports of finding histologic endometriosis in men [31–34], these occurred in men with prostatic carcinoma undergoing high-dose estrogen therapy. The endometriosis was noted in the tissue specimen at the time of prostatectomy and likely represents hypertrophy of the prostatic utricle, the remnant of the Müllerian duct system in males.

2) Endometriosis is confined to women of reproductive age. One would anticipate that metaplasia would increase with age and hence a metaplastic

etiology does not explain the observed age distribution. In fact, the disease process itself is abruptly halted by the decline in gonadal hormones at the climacteric. A process of estrogen-induced metaplasia could explain these findings, but a hormonal requirement for metaplasia has yet to be demonstrated.

3) "Endometriosis only comes from endometrium." The requirement for the presence of endometrial tissue within the uterus to develop this disease is a universal observation. This further implies that endometrium represents the source of cells contributing to the development of the ectopic implants. While cases of "Müllerian agenesis" have been associated with endometriosis, there is rarely a situation in which a portion of the Müllerian duct is not present. Typically, the fallopian tubes are present, as well as a small blind uterine horn at the medial aspect of the tube providing the source of endometrial cells [35].

4) Ectopic endometrial implants are not uniformly distributed within the peritoneum. If metaplasia represents the pathophysiologic process for development of the disease, one would have anticipated a fairly uniform distribution on peritoneal surfaces. As the vast majority of the disease is present in the pelvis, this is inconsistent with the celomic metaplastic hypothesis.

5) The anatomic pattern of endometriosis does not follow the distribution of the celomic membrane. As Maximov [36] and Filatow [37] demonstrated that the celomic membrane contributes both to the peritoneal cavity and the lining of the thoracic cavity, one would anticipate endometriosis would be present in the chest as well. Endometriosis has rarely been reported in the chest, inconsistent with the embryologic distribution of the celomic membrane.

Considering the above issues as well as the lack of experimental evidence demonstrating that the celomic membrane can undergo metaplasia in the adult, it appears that the celomic metaplasia theory of development of endometriosis has virtually no supporting scientific evidence. This concept appears to be only of historical interest, without justification for concluding it plays any role in the development of endometriosis by current standards of scientific inquiry.

Another possible etiology is the stimulation of embryonic rests of Müllerian origin. The anatomic distribution of endometriosis, however, does not follow the path of the Müllerian (paramesonephric) duct system and consequently there is virtually nothing to support that concept.

Our modern day understanding of endometriosis began with the pioneering efforts of a private practitioner, Dr. J.A. Sampson, in Albany, New York.

Through a series of publications, he proposed a theory for the development of endometriosis that has had substantial clinical and scientific support [38–54]. Sampson proposed that the menstrual effluent contained viable endometrial cells of both the stromal and glandular elements, which could be transplanted to ectopic sites. Several routes of dissemination have been observed including lymphatic, vascular, and iatrogenic dissemination as well as a retrograde menstruation. The latter, however, probably represents the route of dissemination of endometrial cells in the vast majority of patients whose disease is confined to the peritoneal surfaces of the pelvic peritoneum and viscera present in the pelvis. Sampson's concepts aroused tremendous controversy, and despite his considerable efforts, Sampson did not receive accolades for his work, but rather it was much maligned for criticizing the dogma of celomic metaplasia. Even to the present, most practitioners of obstetrics and gynecology lack a comprehensive understanding of this disease process.

Lymphatic Dissemination

Endometrium spread outside the uterus by lymphatic drainage was first suggested by Halban, in 1924, when he reported five women with endometriosis thought to have spread their disease via the lymphatics [55]. It was not until 1949, however, that Javert presented unequivocal histologic evidence of endometrial tissue in lymphatic channels and lymph nodes [56]. Two additional reports further substantiate this mode of dissemination. The first is that of endometriosis in the umbilicus, which is known to be a drainage site of lymphatics of pelvic origin [57] and the second being the report of an adenoacanthoma in an endometriotic cyst from an obturator lymph node [58]. This appears to be a relatively rare route of dissemination.

Hematogenous Dissemination

In 1925, Sampson suggested vascular transport as a route of dissemination of endometrium to distant sites [45]. As with the situation with lymphatic dissemination, Javert presented unequivocal histologic evidence of endometrial tissue within pelvic veins supporting this concept [56]. Despite a very low frequency of hematogenous spread, there are multiple cases of endometriosis reported in the lung, skin, thigh, and extremities to illustrate this mode of transport [30,55,59–64].

Iatrogenic Dissemination

Inadvertently spreading endometrial cells at the time of surgery has long been anecdotally observed by gynecologists [30]. Experimentally transplanting endometrium has also been accomplished, further supporting this infrequent mode of transplantation [65].

Retrograde Menstruation

After observing the pattern of endometriosis for many years, Sampson concluded that endometrial cells regurgitated through the fallopian tubes at the time of menstruation explained the vast majority of endometriosis he observed. Through a series of insightful observations he refined his concept, and it represented the main challenge to the theory of celomic metaplasia. This is a clear concise record of scientific observation and remains as the substantial body of supporting data to this day.

In trying to understand the retrograde menstrual process, it is important that the physiology of the normal menstrual cycle be well understood. While each species differs in its strategy for reproduction, cyclic ovarian changes culminating in ovulation occur in virtually all mammalian species. In most animals, coitus or the presence of a conceptus is required to develop a luteal phase and delay another cycle of follicular recruitment. In human and subhuman primates, however, spontaneous luteal phases occur in the absence of coitus or a conceptus. Unique histologic and functional changes in the endometrium, i.e., secretory endometrium with decidualization[66], occur in response to progesterone being secreted in large quantities by the corpus luteum. Presumably, progestational action triggers the series of biochemical events necessary to prepare the genital tract for early embryo growth and development as well as neovascularization once implantation has taken place.

When pregnancy occurs, the fetal signal, human chorionic gonadotropin (hCG), provides trophic support to the corpus luteum, maintaining its lifespan. In the absence of a conceptus, the luteal changes must revert to the proliferative pattern associated with follicular recruitment for the subsequent cycle. The corpus luteum undegoes a predictable regression with declining progesterone production terminating in menstruation. Menses involves a collapse in endometrial height, reversal of the histologic changes in the endometrium, and shedding of a modest number of endometrial cells along with tissue fluid and blood [3,66].

The biochemical events that control menstruation are intimately involved with uterine prostaglandin production [67]. Endometrial tissue gains the ability to synthesize prostaglandins late in the luteal phase commensurate with morphologic decidualization of the endometrial stroma. The balance between vasodilating and vasconstricting prostaglandins shifts toward vasoconstriction, causing the spiral arterioles supplying the superficial layers of endometrium to go into spasm. This results in tissue hypoxia, ischemia, and autolysis. Blood, extracellular fluid, and cells are shed and comprise the menstrual effluent [3,66]. Careful examination of the cellular content of menses demonstrates that the cell loss is predominantly clusters and individual cells rather than intact fragments of endometrium [3].

Under the influence of prostaglandins, the adjacent myometrium undergoes rhythmic contractions, elevating the pressure within the uterus and expelling the menses [67]. There are three possible routes of egress of the menstrual effluent, the cervix and both fallopian tubes. Obviously, the cervical canal has a larger diameter than the oviducts and presumably the least resistance, affording the greatest volume of menstrual flow in that direction. Little is known, however, of the physiology of the uterotubal junction with respect to preventing regurgitation of menstrual debris, particularly under the influence of the changes in prostaglandin synthesis during menses.

Some menstrual regurgitation must occur almost universally, as evidenced by bloody peritoneal dialysates at the time of menses [68] and hemorrhagic peritoneal fluid retrieved at laparoscopy during menses [69,70]. Impediments to uterine outflow either on a congenital basis or after surgical manipulation are well known to predispose to the development of endometriosis. The explanation is probably the volume of regurgitated menstrual debris. When no significant pathology exists, the pressure relationships between the cervix and fallopian tubes likely determine the proportion of menses that is regurgitated, but little is known of the determinants of directional flow of menstrual effluent. Interestingly, women with short cycle lengths and menses for a week or longer have been reported to have greater than twice the risk of developing endometriosis [71].

If retrograde menstruation is to be the explanation for the bulk of pelvic endometriosis observed, there are three basic principles that must be supported by scientific data. First, viable endometrial cells must enter the peritoneal cavity through the fallopian tubes. Second, cells within the menstrual debris can indeed find conditions suitable for transplantation on pelvic structures. Lastly, the anatomic distribution of the disease should fit the principles of transplantation biology for exfoliated cells present in the pelvic cavity.

The evidence to support the entry of viable endometrial cells through the fallopian tubes is as follows:

1) The presence of viable endometrial cells in the menstrual debris has been demonstrated by culturing the menstrual effluent and obtaining tissue cultures of endometrial cells [72,73].

2) The presence of endometrial cells in the fallopian tube has been demonstrated by perfusing excised human oviducts [74].

3) The presence of endometrial cells in the peritoneal cavity has been demonstrated by cytologic evaluation of peritoneal fluid obtained through culdocentesis [75].

4) Retrograde menstruation has been demonstrated, as noted earlier, to be a near universal event to some degree.

Evidence to support the ability of endometrial cells to be transplanted includes:

1) Endometrial tissue can implant and grow within the peritoneal cavity as demonstrated in a variety of animal species [76].

2) Neither of the two dominant ovarian steroids (estrogen or progesterone) are required for implantation or early growth of endometrial cells. There appears to be some long-term necessity for these hormones to maintain viable endometrial implants [77].

3) Endometrial cells obtained from the menstrual effluent have been demonstrated to be transplantable to abdominal wall fascia [30,65].

Evidence that endometrial tissue in the peritoneal cavity implants in a pattern consistent with the tenets of the transplantation of biology includes:

1) Endometriosis is extremely common at the site of entry in the peritoneal cavity, i.e., the fallopian tube ostia [78]. Under natural circumstances the oviductal ostia are located near the uterosacral ligament at the base of the broad ligament, an extremely common site of endometrial cell implantation.

2) Transplantation of free-floating endometrial cells in the peritoneal cavity appears to be influenced by the effects of gravity within the abdomen. Regardless of whether women are sitting, standing, or lying, the pelvic cavity is the most dependent portion of the abdomen and little upper abdominal endometriosis is observed. With uterine anteflexion, the pelvis is divided into anterior and posterior compartments with the anterior one being the uterovesical fold and the posterior one being the posterior cul-de-sac. With that uterine position, implants are relatively equally distributed between compartments. With a retroflexed uterus there is no dependent anterior compartment, and the disease distribution under those circumstances shifts predominantly to the posterior compartment (Table I) [78].

3) Mobile pelvic structures would be less likely to allow attachment of transplanted endometrial cells, whereas fixed structures would be anticipated to have a higher frequency of implants. This prediction is consistent with the observation that the fallopian tubes and small bowel (actively mobile struc-

TABLE I. Influence of Uterine Position on the Distribution of Endometriosis in 187 Women Undergoing Laparoscopy for Infertility [78]

Uterine position	Anterior compartment endometriosis[a] (%)	Posterior compartment endometriosis[b] (%)
Anteflexion (n=118)	43.3	58.4
Midposition (n=18)	38.9	61.1
Retroflexed (n=51)	11.8	88.2

[a]Anterior compartment endometriosis is defined by the presence of endometrial implants anterior to the uterus in the uterovesicle fold or on the peritoneum overlying the bladder.
[b]Posterior compartment endometriosis is defined by the presence of endometrial implants posterior to the uterus in the cul-de-sac, on the posterior broad ligament, or on the ovaries.

tures) are involved with endometriosis far less often than the nonmobile ovary, pelvic peritoneum, and the fixed portion of the sigmoid colon [78].

4) Transplantation should be influenced by local tissue factors such as the suitability of the surface epithelium, vascularity, and hormone production. The peritoneum overlying the pelvic viscera as well as the pelvic side-wall represents a favorable site for implantation, being one cell layer thick with good vascularization. This is particularly in contrast with the squamous epithelium lining the lower genital tract, which is regularly exposed to endometrial cells during menses yet is an infrequent site of involvement. As endometrial tissue is dependent upon ovarian hormone production for growth, it would be anticipated that the ovary would represent an optimal site of implantation. Additionally, the proximity to the tubal ostia and the corresponding contour of the ovarian capsule should enhance cell attachment. It is not surprising, then, that the ovary represents the most common single site of involvement with endometriosis [4,21,78–80].

After reviewing the above data, it becomes obvious that the preponderence of evidence suggests that endometriosis is a consequence of transplantation of viable endometrial cells regurgitated through the fallopian tubes at the time of menses. In establishing the etiology for this disease, it is appropriate to consider Koch's postulates as modified for endometriosis. These appear to have been fulfilled, defining the pathophysiologic link between a retrograde menstruation and the observed entity. First, endometriosis is defined as the presence of cells morphologically identical to normal endometrium at an ectopic site. Second, the ectopic implants respond to reproductive hormones. Third, endometriosis can be recreated by iatrogenically transplanting endometrium. Under natural conditions a route of entry for endometrial cells into the peritoneal cavity is well established. Finally, experimentally created endometriosis is histologically identical to that occurring under natural circumstances. Although the dissemination of viable endometrial cells by other routes may rarely occur, the vast preponderance of endometriosis can be accounted for by retrograde menstruation as described by the insightful efforts of Sampson over 50 years ago.

PATHOLOGY

Macroscopic Appearance

Clinicians have long diagnosed the presence of endometriosis by the characteristics blue-gray "powder burn" lesions on peritoneal surfaces over the pelvic peritoneum or pelvic viscera. This distinctive appearance can be attributed to the encapsulation of menstrual debris, indicating the menstrual cyclicity of the implants. Upon excision of these lesions, the discoloration frequently disappears as the encapsulation is incised and the liquid debris is inadvertently lost, making identification of the lesion for accurate histologic sectioning difficult. As a consequence, routine histologic examination often fails to reveal widely scattered endometrial glands and stroma in a background of collagen disposition. Consequently, the diagnosis is frequently more adequately made by the operating surgeon than the pathologist exclusively viewing histologic material.

The gross appearance of ectopic endometrium is not limited to the classic "powder burn," and the appearance is critically dependent upon the longevity of the process. The earliest sign that retrograde menstruation has resulted in transplantation of endometrial cells is hemosiderin staining of the peritoneal surfaces in dependent places in the pelvis. Within that background, viable cells may implant and the initial appearance may be any irregularity or discoloration of the peritoneal surface. Initially, these lesions may appear hemorrhagic or tan in color. After establishment of a viable endometrial transplant, menstrual shedding of the implant initiates a localized inflammatory reaction. In response, the scarification process begins and once this has completely enclosed the implants (Fig. 1), the entrapped menstrual debris gives the lesion the typical blue-gray "powder burn" appearance. If the inflammatory process obliterates or devascularizes the endometrial cells, eventually this discoloration disappears, and a white plaque of old collagen is all that remains of the ectopic implant.

Scarring of the peritoneum around endometrial implants is the typical finding. In addition to encapsulating an isolated implant, the scar may deform the surrounding peritoneum or result in the development of adhesions between adjacent pelvic viscera. Pelvic adhesions due to endometriosis are

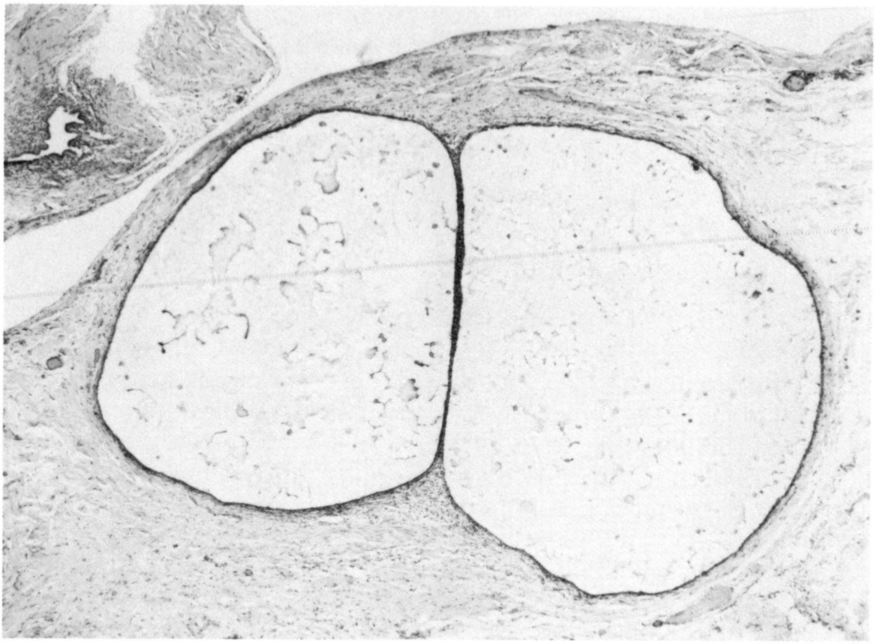

Fig. 1. A peritoneal implant of endometriosis. A typical blue-grey "powder burn" lesion on the peritoneal surface is present with dilated endometrial glands surrounded by an ill-defined stroma and a marked fibrotic reaction (H&E, 40×).

most common between immobile pelvic structures which are in natural apposition within the pelvis (Table II). Adhesions with endometriosis are found commonly between 1) the posterior leaf of the broad ligament and the ovary, 2) the anterior bladder peritoneum and the visceral peritoneum over the anterior aspect of the uterus, and 3) the dependent sigmoid colon and the posterior aspect of the vagina and cervix. The fallopian tubes and small bowel are most often spared, as their mobility reduces the likelihood of contact with peritoneal implants with sufficient regularity to prevent establishment of an intervening collagen matrix. Intratubal endometriosis causing uterotubal obstruction represents approximately one-third of the cases of proximal tubal occlusion [81]. The finding of intraluminal scarring in the contralateral tube suggests the collagen deposition is the end result of reaction to menstrual shedding within the isthmic segment of the fallopian tube. Whether the collagen deposition is secondary to the irritant effect of menstruation or a more specific secretory product of endometrium is unclear, but

TABLE II. Distribution of Endometriosis and Adhesions by Site in 187 Women Undergoing Laparoscopy for Infertility[78]

	Endometriosis			Adhesions		
Site	Left	(%)	Right	Left	(%)	Right
Ovary	44.0		31.3	24.7		14.3
Anterior utero vesicle fold		34.6			2.2	
Posterior cul-de-sac		34.0			11.0	
Posterior broad ligament	25.2		21.4	27.5		16.5
Uterosacral ligament	20.8		15.3	4.4		2.7
Uterus		11.5			3.3	
Fallopian tube	4.3		1.6	15.4		11.0
Sigmoid colon		3.8			12.1	
Ureter	1.1		1.6	—		—
Anterior broad ligament	0.0		1.1	1.6		1.1
Small bowel		0.5			2.2	
Anterior bladder peritoneum		0.5			0.5	
Round ligament	0.5		0.5	1.1		1.1

the former is more likely as there is virtually no intrauterine scarring during normal menstruation.

The extent of scarring may vary dramatically from patient to patient and even on one organ the degree of scarring may be quite variable. For example, when endometriosis is present under the ovarian capsule, large endometrial cysts may form in a totally free and mobile ovary (Fig. 2). By contrast, when small endometrial implants are present on the ovarian capsule, dense adhesions to the posterior leaf of the broad ligament or the sigmoid colon are the rule (Fig. 3). Extension of the scar surrounding implants to retroperitoneal organs is occasionally observed. There is usually little functional compromise of large organs such as the bladder and bowel despite extensive involvement with endometriosis. The ureter, by contrast, with its small caliber is more vulnerable to obstruction due to scar contracture [82]. Its course under the peritoneal surface near the fallopian tube ostia may contribute to the higher incidence of functional compromise of the urinary system than the gastrointestinal tract. Medical suppressive therapy designed to interrupt ovarian function and shrink the implants will be ineffective if the problem is related to scar contracture rather than cycling endometrial cells within the implant.

Anatomic Distribution

As noted earlier, the anatomic distribution of endometrial implants can be predicted by the simple principles of transplant biology. The pattern of

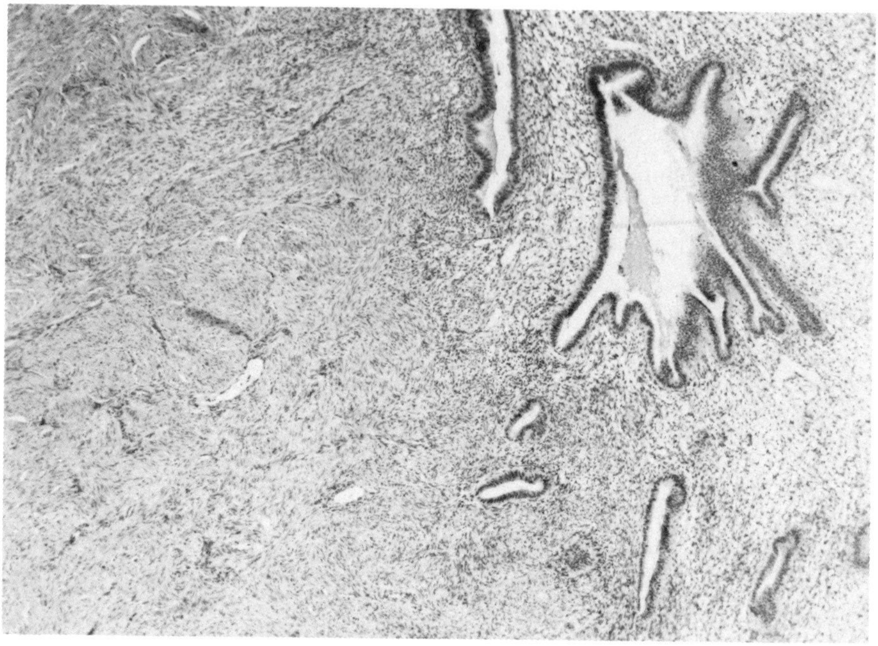

Fig. 2. Ovarian endometriosis. Endometrial glands and stroma are present within the ovarian stroma. Note the minimal collagen deposition surrounding the lesion and the relatively high density of glands (H&E, 52×).

disease may be influenced by the patient selection criteria. Patients presenting with pelvic pain may well have a different pattern of disease from those complaining of infertility. Table II depicts a recent study of the pattern of endometriosis in a population of infertility patients [78]. The ovary is the most frequently involved because of its unique characteristics. The next most likely sites are the anterior uterovesicle fold and the posterior cul-de-sac, presumably governed by the effects of gravity. The next most common sites are the posterior aspect of the broad ligament and uterosacral ligaments. Proximity to the tubal ostia probably accounts for the high frequency of disease at these sites. Of the pelvic viscera, the uterus is most commonly affected due to its immobility. The fallopian tube and sigmoid colon follow the uterus in frequency, and the small bowel with its active peristalsis is far less frequently involved. While these findings differ slightly from the anatomic distribution of endometriosis observed in earlier studies at laparotomy, the ovary remains the most commonly involved pelvic structure regardless of the presenting symptomatology.

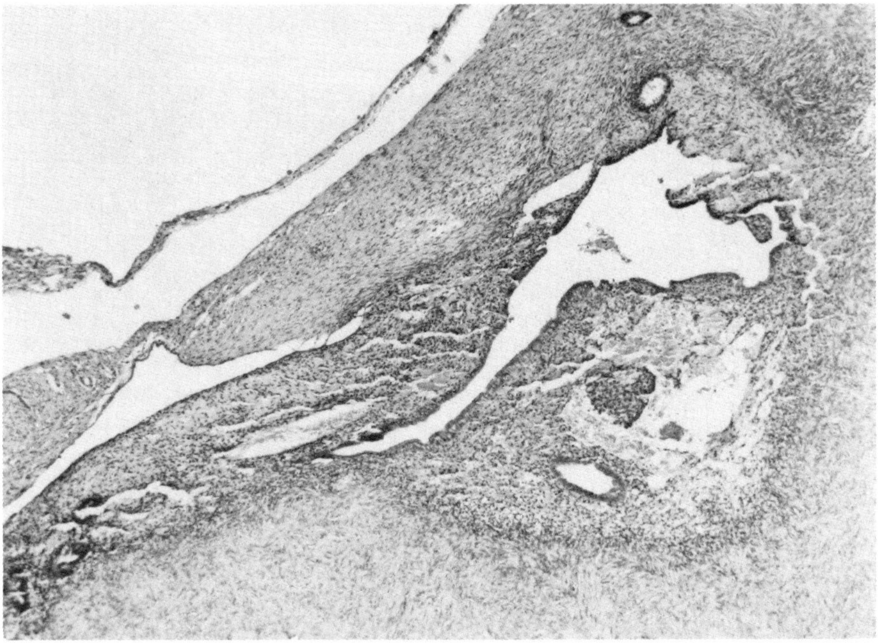

Fig. 3. A surface ovarian implant. An endometrial implant on the capsule of the ovary. There is evidence of hemorrhage in the stroma surrounding the gland as well as vascularized adhesions (H&E, 52×).

Microscopic Appearance

Ever since the original pathologic description of endometriosis, the disease has been defined by the presence of endometrial glands and stroma in an ectopic site. The presence of hemosiderin-laden macrophages (Fig. 4) was used as an indicator of menstrual cyclicity, and this triad of findings has been propagated as the minimum requirements that could unequivocally demonstrate the presence of ectopic endometrium. This was felt to take precedence over the gross appearance, location, or clinical presentation of the disease. Unfortunately, this pathological approach does not take into consideration the dynamic pathophysiologic process endometriosis represents, but is rather an attempt to define criteria by which the disease can be unequivocally identified. As the classic "powder burn" lesions may not possess all these characteristics, the disease will be significantly underdiagnosed utilizing these overly stringent and unvalidated criteria.

It is unusual to find endometriotic implants with a histologic pattern identical to that of normal endometrium [83]. This is not surprising in view

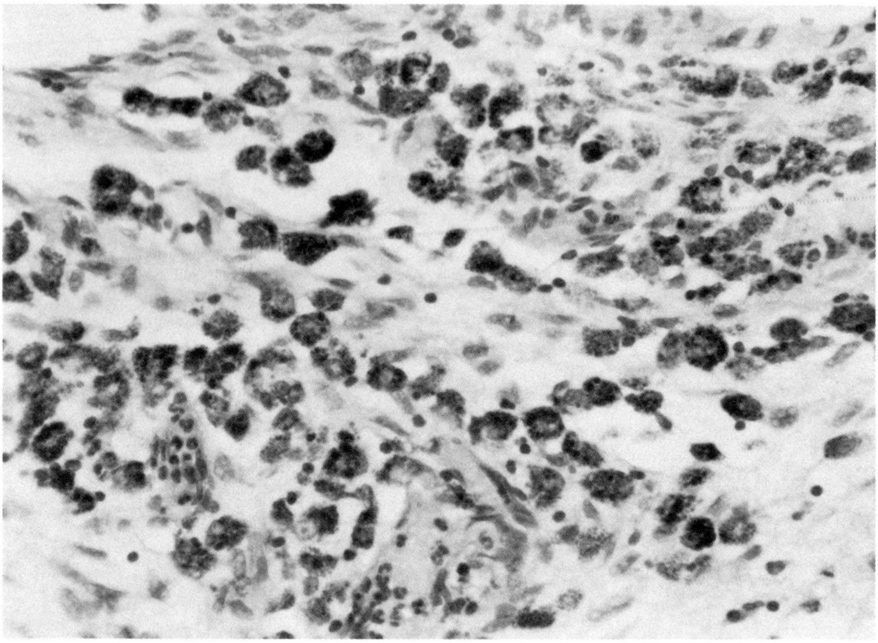

Fig. 4. Hemosiderin-laden macrophages. This high-power photomicrograph was taken from an area surrounding an endometrial implant and the hemosiderin-laden macrophages provide evidence of chronic hemorrhage, presumably menstrual cyclicity (H&E, 325×).

of the fact that menstruation involves the loss of isolated cells or clusters of cells rather than intact fragments of endometrium [3]. The typical endometrial lesion reflects this pattern of cell shedding, being composed of isolated endometrial glandular components with or without some adjacent stroma (Fig. 5). These glands frequently become cystic, as they lack the appropriate gland ostia for dispensing secretory material as well as menstrual debris. This further distorts their architecture, making their identification as endometrial in origin difficult. Endometriosis may be confused with mesonephric remnants, inflammatory changes, or reactive peritoneal inclusion cysts. The muscular wall of mesonephric remnants can easily be distinguished with connective tissue strains, which may be necessary on occasion. Endometrial stroma is particularly difficult to identify, because the individual stromal cells are frequently indistinguishable from surrounding fibroblasts. Thus identification of isolated stromal implants has not been reported, but undoubtedly occurs.

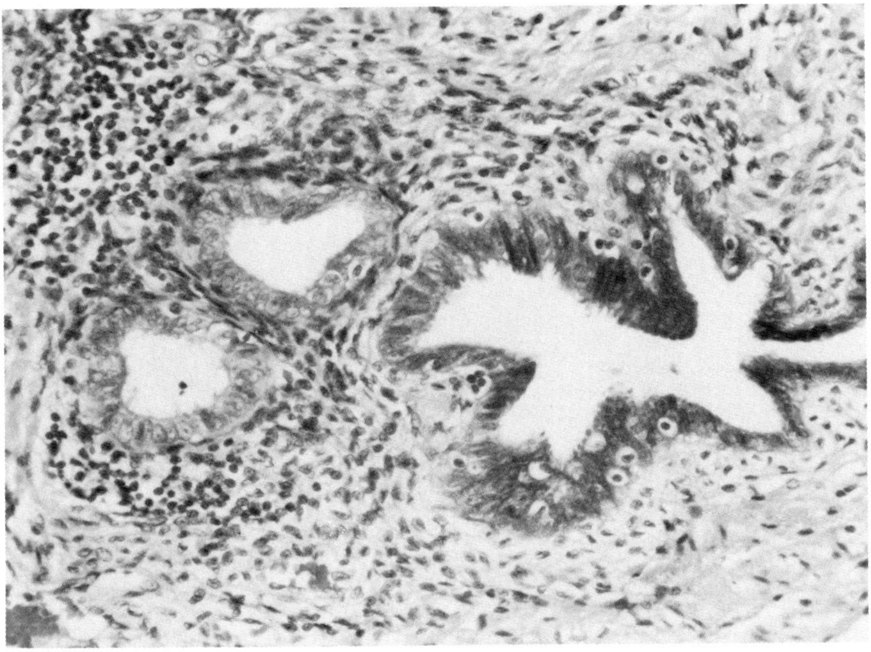

Fig. 5. A peritoneal endometrial implant. The endometrial glands in this lesion are surrounded by a nondescript cellular background without specific characteristics identifying it as endometrial stroma. Distinction between the fibroblastic proliferation and endometrial stromal cells is virtually impossible (H&E, 250×).

The ovary represents a relatively unique site of implantation, as the levels of gonadal steroids surpass those in the circulation, and hence this represents an ideal environment for implantation and endometrial growth (Fig. 2). Superficial implants of endometriosis on the ovary resemble implants at other peritoneal sites (Fig. 3). In contrast, when endometrial cells enter the ovarian stroma, large endometrial cysts may form that are filled with a viscous chocolate-colored liquid, i.e., "chocolate cysts" or endometrioma, which represent debris from cyclic menstruation [38–42]. These may attain impressive size and completely obliterate the normal ovary. There is usually a well-demarcated separation between the endometrial cyst wall and the normal adjacent ovarian stroma. The epithelial lining of the endometrioma may initially have resembled the endometrium, but with continued menstrual cyclicity without drainage of the menstrual material, pressure atrophy compresses the epithelium into a flat cuboidal pattern without specific distinguishing characteristics (Fig. 6). Under these circumstances the histologic

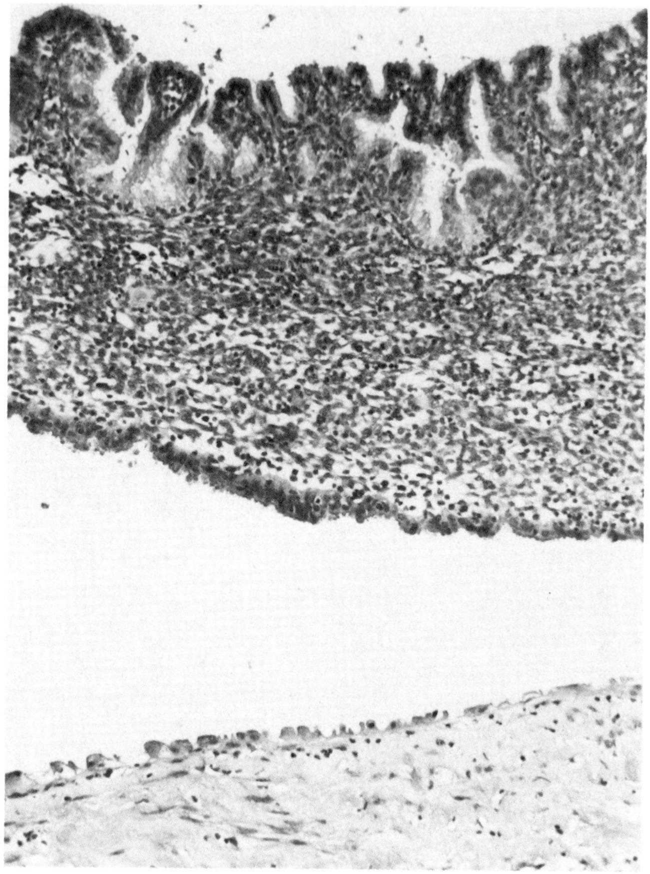

Fig. 6. The wall of an ovarian endometrioma. Note the variable appearance of the walls of this "chocolate cyst." The histology ranges from an atrophied epithelium to virtually normal endometrial glandular formation (H&E, 170×).

appearance may be of no diagnostic help except in the exclusion of malignancy.

The entry of endometrial cells into the ovarian stroma has long been a source of controversy. The answer probably lies with the events surrounding ovulation. The corpus luteum with its ovulatory stigma represents a break in the ovarian capsule with excellent vascular supply and high production of gonadal steroids. The ovulatory stigma represents an optimal site for implantation, and with rapid reepithelialization of the capsule, the endometrial implant is quickly confined within the ovarian stroma.

Ultrastructural Appearance

Electron microscopy has been useful in investigating the physiologic events of the menstrual cycle. Normal endometrium undergoes a series of ultrastructural changes paralleling the histologic changes [84,85]. Characteristic changes include the appearance of giant mitochondria and nuclear channel systems coincident with ovulation. While not exhaustively studied, endometrial implants do not demonstrate these characteristic ultrastructural changes of normal endometrium [86]. The presence of collagen surrounding the implants is readily confirmed by identification of the collagen fibrils, and endometrial stromal cells can be identified by this means even within a background of scarification [86]. A fascinating recent finding has been the identification by high-resolution electron microscopy of endometrial cells loosely attached to the peritoneal surface on grossly normal peritoneum when endometriosis is present elsewhere in the pelvis [87]. This suggests that a much larger number of endometrial cells are present in the peritoneum than actually develop into grossly apparent lesions. Further data should be forthcoming regarding the environmental requirements of implantation.

Secretory Function of Endometrial Implants

Paralleling the histologic changes in the menstrual cycle, a sequence of biochemical events occur designed to either provide an environment conducive to embryo implantation or, in the absence of conception, to undergo menses and revert the endometrium to the proliferative pattern. Using qualitative histochemistry, the microscopic changes present in endometrium have been observed in ectopic implants [88]. In the absence of pregnancy, the decidualization of endometrium coincides with the ability to produce prostaglandins, and these have been identified in ectopically implanted endometrium [89]. Prostanoid concentrations in the peritoneal fluid of women with endometriosis have been extensively investigated with many studies demonstrating elevations [90–96], although others were unable to confirm these observations [97–100]. There are problems with many of these studies that are inherent with the use of prostaglandins as markers of endometrial secretory activity. Prostagandin production is cycle-dependent, their half-life is short, and other cells within the peritoneal cavity, i.e., peritoneal macrophages, synthesize them so they are not specific for endometriosis. Prolactin, another decidual secretory product, has also been used as an endometrial marker with some advantages over prostanoids. It is a large protein and, hence, its half-life in blood is substantially longer and it is not known to have another source within the abdomen. When evaluated carefully in a cycle-dependent fashion, prolactin was not found elevated in the peritoneal fluid of women with endometriosis [101]. As a consequence of these considerations, it is still unclear whether endometrial implants have sufficient secretory capability to influence the biochemistry of the peritoneal fluid.

Hormonal Responsiveness of Endometrial Implants

The fact that endometrial implants can undergo cyclic histologic changes similar to those found with normal endometrium demonstrates that ectopic endometrium responds to gonadal hormones. Quantitation of this response, however, is difficult to evaluate, owing to the small amounts of tissue present at ectopic sites. As noted earlier, the majority of implants do not demonstrate synchronous histologic changes with the comparable uterine endometrium [83]. The reason for this is not known but may include deficient steroid receptor populations, altered epithelial-stromal relationships, the influence of the surrounding scarification process, or pressure atrophy from the inability to extrude secretory products through gland ostia.

The requirement for gonadal hormones to maintain endometrium seems clear. Castration, menopause, pregnancy, or therapeutic suppression of gonadal function can dramatically alter the pattern of disease. Under an altered hormonal environment, endometrial atrophy occurs, either directly because of hormone deprivation or after decidual atrophy with the high levels of estrogen and progesterone associated with pregnancy.

Investigations into the presence of steroid receptors in ectopic endometrial implants has been hampered by the small number of glandular and stromal cells within the implant as well as the heterogeneity of tissue with substantial amounts of intervening collagen. While most implants can be demonstrated to possess progesterone receptors, only 30% have estrogen receptors [102]. Even on the ovary where the gonadal steroid milieu is high, implants have far fewer estrogen and progesterone receptors than normal epithelium [103,104]. A thorough understanding of the stromal-epithelial relationship in terms of hormonal responsiveness of normal endometrium is still lacking. Similarly, when autoradiograms are used to qualitatively assess estrogen receptors, there seems to be substantial differences between the distribution of receptors in the stroma and glands of ectopic implants of endometrium [105]. As a normal stromal-epithelial relationship is probably necessary to generate a histologic response to a rapidly fluctuating hormonal environment, it is not surprising that there is substantial variability in the histologic appearance of ectopic endometrium.

The endocrine requirements for implantation are unknown. Based on nonhuman primate experiments, it appears steroids are not required for the early transplantation events but are necessary for continued viability and certainly for cyclic histologic and secretory changes [77]. As the peritoneal fluid contains high levels of gonadal hormones [106] which fluctuate during the menstrual cycle, free-floating endometrial cells are exposed to these steroids. An alteration from the normal histologic cyclicity would then probably be due to other factors such as receptor levels, stromal-epithelial relationships, or local tissue factors such as vascularity, collagen deposition, and inflammatory changes.

Influence of Endometriosis on Peritoneal Fluid

It has become apparent recently that the presence of endometriosis is associated with changes in the peritoneal fluid volume, leukocyte population, and biochemistry. This can most accurately be characterized as the presence of an intraperitoneal inflammatory exudate. While there is some cyclic fluctuation in the volume of peritoneal fluid in normal women without endometriosis, the volume of peritoneal fluid has generally been elevated in women with endometriosis [107,108] and even cases of ascites have been reported [109–112]. The nonneoplastic cell populations within the peritoneal fluid have generally been interpreted by cytopathologists as "reactive mesothelial cells." Based on their functional characteristics, however, these cells appear to be predominantly mononuclear phagocytes. With standard differential cell-counting using Giemsa staining, the population is composed of approximately 90% mononuclear phagocytes, i.e., macrophages, with a small number of lymphocytes and polymorphonuclear leukocytes [108]. The macrophages stain positively for nonspecific esterase and peroxidase [108], phagocytize polysytrene beads [113], lyse tumor cells [114], and can have phagocytosis opsinized by antibody coating of the target cells [115,116].

The total macrophage counts are dramatically higher when endometriosis is present [108] and, based on the percentage of cells staining for proteolytic enzymes [117], these cells are activated. Even in women without endometriosis, obstruction of the fallopian tube reduces the number of leukocytes present in the peritoneal fluid [113]. Some retrograde menstruation occurs in all women, and this may represent the irritant responsible for the elicitation of this inflammatory response, being exaggerated in women with endometriosis. Higher macrophage populations are also present in the ampullary portion of the fallopian tube in women with endometriosis, paralleling the peritoneal fluid number of leukocytes [113]. They appear to enter from the peritoneal cavity, as when proximal tubal obstruction is present, the cell population correlates with the peritoneal fluid levels. When distal tubal obstruction is present, the leukocyte population within the hydrosalpinx fluid is extremely low in the absence of recent infection [113]. Despite these dramatic changes in the peritoneal fluid, no differences in circulating lymphocyte populations have been identified [118], indicating the localized nature of the inflammatory process.

While the stimulus for this localized inflammatory response cannot be unequivocally determined, it is likely it involves either the presence of menstrual debris arriving in the peritoneal cavity via the oviducts or because of menstrual debris from sloughing implants. As the number of endometrial cells in each implant is very small and typically encapsulated by scar, retrograde menstruation is a far more attractive candidate. In the absence of fever or signs of systemic infection, bacteria entering the pelvic cavity via the lower genital tract is an unlikely cause. Secretory products from the local implants are candidates for eliciting this exudate, but this seems unlikely in view of the absence of a specific decidual protein, prolactin, being elevated in the peritoneal fluid [101].

The biochemistry of the peritoneal fluid in women with endometriosis is also altered. As noted earlier, prostanoid concentrations in peritoneal fluid have been variably reported as elevated as well as increases in proteolytic enzymes [117] consistent with a localized inflammatory reaction. Other enzymes, such as plasminogen activator, are not elevated in peritoneal fluid of women with endometriosis [119], so that situation awaits more clarification.

Immunology of Endometriosis

A major question remaining to be investigated is why some women develop the disease and others with similar reproductive patterns do not. As this disease represents transplantation of normal tissue to an ectopic site, autoimmune phenomena have been implicated [120,121] with the hypothesis that patients with endometriosis have a subtly different immune system allowing the development of the disease. Despite being an active area of investigation, little clinical data in humans are available. Complement deposition has been noted surrounding endometrial glands within the uterus in women who have endometriosis [120]. The implication is that the explanted endometrial tissue stimulates an immune response also detected in the endometrium, which reduces the probability of implantation. Further support of this concept came when Badawy et al. demonstrated the apparent presence of antibodies to endometrial cell antigens [122]. Ouchterlony immunodiffusion produced precipitation lines between autologous endometrial cell homogenates and serum in two of three women with endometriosis, but not in three infertile control women without endometriosis [122]. Similarly, antibodies directed against endometrial antigens were demonstrated by hemoagglutination in 11 of 13 women with endometriosis, but not in any control women [123]. In this study, antibody titers directed against ovarian components (thecal and granulosa cells) were higher in women with endometriosis than normal women, and the two women lacking antibodies to endometrium were the only ones without ovarian involvement of the endometriosis. Concentrations of complement components (C_3c and C_4) were noted to be elevated in the serum and peritoneal fluid of women with endometriosis [122], suggesting a complement-mediated cell injury. Further studies will clearly be needed to evaluate this potential antibody-mediated response in women with endometriosis.

Women with endometriosis have no clinically apparent propensity for autoimmune disease and are in generally good health. Their immune status has been suggested to be altered by the finding that cytotoxicity mediated by T-lymphocytes to autologous endometrial cells in vitro was reduced [124]. This finding correlated inversely with the stage of disease. An altered lifespan of the peritoneal macrophage has recently been suggested as a pathogenetic mechanism for the development of endometriosis [125].

Several studies have investigated the relationship of a membrane antigen, CA-125, in women with endometriosis. This surface antigen is present on a variety of adult and fetal human tissues [126] and has been markedly elevated in the serum of women with ovarian cancer [127]. It has also been modestly elevated in women without malignancies, including women in the first trimester of pregnancy, with acute pelvic inflammatory disease, and after gynecologic surgery [128]. Several reports suggest that serum levels of CA-125 are elevated in women with endometriosis particularly with advanced disease [128–131]. The reason for this elevation remains unclear, but possibilities include a response to a noninfectious inflammatory process or a manifestation of celomic epithelial differentiation. As the antigen has been detected on the peritoneum, the origin of the shed antigen may not represent the endometrial tissue per se but the degree of peritoneal involvement. It does not appear that serum levels of CA-125 will be adequate for the diagnosis of endometriosis or to differentiate it from ovarian cancer.

A great deal of effort will be required to better characterize any purported immunologic differences in women with endometriosis. This is particularly true as the distinction between the effect of endometriosis on the immune system versus a predisposition for the development of endometriosis on an altered immune basis is very difficult to separate.

REFERENCES

1. Aral SO, Cates W Jr: The increasing concern with infertility: why now? Science 250:2327, 1983.

2. Olive DL, Haney AF: Endometriosis - Associated infertility: A critical review of therapeutic approaches. Obstet Gynecol Surv 41:538, 1986.
3. Flowers CE Jr, Wilborn WH: New observations in the physiology of menstruation. Obstet Gynecol 51:16, 1978.
4. Holmes WR: Endometriosis. Am J Gynecol 43:255, 1942.
5. Sensky TE, Liu DTY: Endometriosis: associations with menorrhagia, infertility and oral contraceptives. Int J Gynecol Obstet 17:573, 1980.
6. Norwood GE: Sterility and fertility in women with pelvic endometriosis. Obstet Gynecol 3:456, 1960.
7. Olive DL, Franklin RR, Gratkins LV: Association between endometriosis and spontaneous abortions: a retrospective clinical study. J Reprod Med 27:333, 1982.
8. Huffman W: Endometriosis in young teenage girls. Pediatr Ann 10:44, 1981.
9. Hanton EM, Malkasian GD, Jr, Dockerty MB, et al: Endometriosis in young women. Am J Obstet Gynecol 98:116, 1967.
10. Baker ER, Horger EO, Williamson HO: Congenital atresia of the uterine cervix: two cases. J Reprod Med 27:156, 1982.
11. Schifrin BS, Erez S, Moore JG: Teenage endometriosis. Am J Obstet Gynecol 116:973, 1973.
12. Strathy JH, Molgaard CA, Coulam CG, et al: Endometriosis and infertility: a laparoscopic study of endometriosis among fertile and infertile women. Fertil Steril 38:667, 1982.
13. Chatman DL, Ward AB: Endometriosis in adolescents. J Reprod Med 27:156, 1982.
14. Kempers RD, Dockerty MB, Hunt AB, et al: Significant postmenopausal endometriosis. Surg Gynec Obstet 111:348, 1960.
15. Punnonen R, Klemi P, Nikkanen V: Postmenopausal endometriosis. Eur J Obstet Gynecol Reprod Biol 11:195, 1980.
16. Djursing H, Peterson K, Weberg E: Symptomatic postmenopausal endometriosis. Acta Obstet Gynecol Scand 60:529, 1981.
17. Fallus R, Rosenblum G: Endometriosis: a study of 260 private hospital cases. Am J Obstet Gynecol 39:964, 1940.
18. Jeffcoat TA: "Principles of Gynaecology." London: Butterworth, 1975.
19. Williams TJ, Pratt JH: Endometriosis in 1,000 consecutive celiotomies: incidence and management. Am J Obstet Gynecol 129:245, 1977.
20. Meigs JV: Medical treatment of endometriosis and significance of endometriosis. Surg Gynecol Obstet 89:317, 1949.
21. Scott RB, Telinde RW: External endometriosis: scourge of private patient. Ann Surg 131:697, 1950.
22. Chatman DL: Endometriosis and the black woman. J Reprod Med 16:303, 1976.
23. Miyazawa K: Incidence of endometriosis among Japanese women. Obstet Gynecol 48:407, 1976.
24. Lloyd FP: Endometriosis in the Negro woman. Am J Obstet Gynecol 89:468, 1964.
25. Ranney B: Endometriosis IV. Hereditary tendencies. Obstet Gynecol 37:734, 1971.
26. Malinak LR, Buttram VC Jr, Elias S, et al.: Heritable aspects of endometriosis II. Clinical characteristics of familial endometriosis. Am J Obstet Gynecol 137:332, 1980.
27. Simpson JL, Elias S, Malinak LR, et al.: Heritable aspects of endometriosis. I. Genetic studies. Am J Obstet Gynecol 137:327, 1980.
28. Lamb K, Hoffman RG, Nichols TR: Family trait analysis: a case-control study of 43 women with endometriosis and their best friends. Am J Obstet Gynecol 154:596, 1986.

29. Moen M, Bratlie A, Moen T: Distribution of HLA-antigens among patients with endometriosis. Acta Obstet Gynecol Scand Suppl 123:25, 1984.
30. Ridley JH: The histogenesis of endometriosis: a review of facts and fancies. Obstet Gynecol Survey 23:1, 1968.
31. Melicow MM, Pachter MR: Endometrial carcinoma of the prostatic utricle (uterus masculinus). Cancer 20:1715, 1967.
32. Olikar AF, Harns AE: Endometriosis of the bladder in a male patient. J Urol 106:858, 1971.
33. Pinkert TC, Catlow CE, Straus R: Endometriosis of the urinary bladder in a man with prostatic carcinoma. Cancer 43:1562, 1979.
34. Schrodt GR, Alcorn MD, Ibanez J: Endometriosis of the male urinary system: a case report. J Urol 124:722, 1980.
35. Rosenfeld DL, Lecher BD: Endometriosis in a patient with Rokitansky-Kuster-Hauser syndrome. Am J Obstet Gynecol 139:105, 1981.
36. Maximow A: Uber der Mesthel (Deckzellen der serosen Haute) und die Zellen der sero sen Exsudate. Untersuchungen an entzundetem Gewebe und an Gewebskulturen. Arch Exp Zellforch 4:1, 1927.
37. Filatow D: Uber die Bildung des Anfangsstaddiums bie der Extremitatenentwicklung. Roux Arch, fur Entwicklungsmechnd, Organe 127:776, 1933.
38. Sampson JA: Perforating hemorrhagic (chocolate) cysts of the ovary. Arch Surgery 3:245, 1921.
39. Sampson JA: Ovarian hematomas of endometrial type (perforating hemorrhagic cysts of the ovary) and implantation adenomas of endometrial type. Boston Med Surg J 186:445, 1922.
40. Sampson JA: Life history of ovarian hematomas. Am J Obstet Gynecol 4:451, 1922.
41. Sampson JA: Intestinal adenomas of endometrial type, their importance, and their relation to ovarian hematomas of endometrial type (perforation hemorrhagic cysts of the ovary). Arch Surg 5:217, 1922.
42. Sampson JA: Benign and malignant endometrial implants in the peritoneal cavity and their relation to certain ovarian tumors. Surg Gynecol Obstet 38:287, 1924.
43. Sampson JA: Endometrial carcinoma of the ovary arising in endometrial tissue in that organ. Arch Surg 10:1, 1925.
44. Sampson JA: Inguinal endometriosis (often reported as endometrial tissue in the groin, adenomyoma in the groin, and adenomyoma of the round ligament). Am J Obstet Gynecol 10:462, 1925.
45. Sampson JA: Heterotopic or misplaced endometrial tissue. Am J Obstet Gynecol 10:649, 1925.
46. Sampson JA: Endometriosis of the sac of the right inguinal hernia associated with pelvic peritoneal endometriosis and endometrial cyst of the ovary. Am J Obstet Gynecol 12:459, 1926.
47. Sampson JA: Metastatic of embolic endometriosis due to menstrual dissemination of endometrial tissue into the venous circulation. Am J Pathol 3:93, 1927.
48. Sampson JA: Peritoneal endometriosis due to the menstrual dissemination of endometrial tissue into the peritoneal cavity. Am J Obstet Gynecol 14:422, 1927.
49. Sampson JA: Endometriosis following salpingectomy. Am J Obstet Gynecol 16:461, 1928.
50. Sampson JA: Infected endometrial cysts of the ovaries: a report of three cases, two of which were bilateral. Am J Obstet Gynecol 18:1, 1929.

51. Sampson JA: Postsalpingectomy endometriosis (endosalpingiosis). Am J Obstet Gynecol 20:443, 1930.
52. Samspon JA: Pelvic endometriosis and tubal fimbriae. Am J Obstet Gynecol 24:497, 1932.
53. Sampson JA: The development of the implantation theory for the origin of peritoneal endometriosis. Am J Obstet Gynecol 40:549, 1940.
54. Sampson JA: Pathogenesis of postsalpingectomy endometriosis in laparotomy scars. Am J Obstet Gynecol 59:596, 1945.
55. Halbin J: Hysateroadenosis metastatica, Die lymphoqere genese der sog, Adenofibromatosis heterotopica. Arch Gynak 124:457, 1925.
56. Javert CT: The spread of benign and malignant endometrium in the lymphatic system with a note of coexisting vascular involvement. Am J Obstet Gynecol 64:780, 1952.
57. Scott RB, Nowak RJ, Tindale RM: Umbilical endometriosis and Cullen's sign: study of lymphatic transport from pelvis to umbilicus in monkeys. Obstet Gynecol 11:556, 1958.
58. Koss IG: Miniature adenocanthoma arising in an adenometriotic cyst in an obturator lymph node. Cancer 16:1369, 1963.
59. Duncan C, Pitney WR: Endometrial tumors in the extremities. Med J Aust 2:175, 1949.
60. Nunn LL: Endometrioma of the thigh. Northwest Med 48:474, 1949.
61. Lattes R, Shepard F, Tovell H, et al.: A clinical and pathologic study of endometriosis of the lung. Surg Gynecol Obstet 103, 552:1956.
62. Rodman MH, Jones CW: Catemenial Hemoptysis due to bronchial endometriosis. NEJH 266:805, 1962.
63. Kitchin JD: Endometriosis, p. 1. In Sciarra JJ (ed): "Gynecology and Obstetrics," Vol. 1. Chapter 20. Philadelphia: Harper & Row, 1982.
64. Javert CT: Pathogenesis of endometriosis based on endometrial homeoplasia direct extension, exfoliation and implantation, lymphomatic and hematogeneous metastasis. Cancer 2:399, 1949.
65. Ridley JH, Edwards IK: Experimental endometriosis in the human. Am J Obstet Gynecol 76:783, 1958.
66. Markee JE: Morphological basis for menstrual bleeding. Bull NY Acad Med 24:253, 1948.
67. Vijayakumar R, Walters WAW: Myometrial prostaglandins during the human menstrual cycle. Am J Obstet Gynecol 141:313, 1981.
68. Blumenkrantz MJ, Glallagher N, Bashore RA, et al: Retrograde menstruation in women undergoing chronic peritoneal dialysis. Obstet Gynecol 57:667, 1981.
69. Halme J, Hammond MG, Hulka JF, et al.: Retrograde menstruation in healthy women and in patients with endometriosis. Obstet Gynecol 64:151, 1984.
70. Liu DTY, Hitchcock A: Endometriosis: its association with retrograde menstruation, dysmenorrhea and tubal pathology. Br J Obstet Gynecol 93:859, 1986.
71. Cramer DW, Wilson E, Stillman RJ, Berger MJ, Belisle S, Schiff I, Albrecht B, Gibson M, Stadel BV, Schoenbaum SC: The relation of endometriosis to menstrual characteristics, smoking, and exercise. JAMA 255:1904, 1986.
72. Cron RS, Gey G: The viability of the cast-off menstrual endometrium. Am J Obstet Gynecol 43:645, 1927.
73. Kistner RW, Wiegler AM, Behrman SJ: Suggested classification for endometriosis: relationship to infertility. Fertil Steril 28:1008, 1977.
74. Geist SH: The viability of fragments of menstrual endometrium. Am J Obstet Gynecol 25:751, 1979.

75. Manning JO, Shaver EF Jr: The demonstration of endometrial cells by Papanicolaou and supravital techniques obtained by culdocentesis. Bull Tulane Univ Med Fac 18:193, 159.
76. Allen E, Peterson LF, Campbell ZB: Clinical and experimental endometriosis. Am J Obstet Gynecol 68:356, 1954.
77. Dizerega GS, Barber DL, Hodgen GD: Endometriosis: role of ovarian steroids in initiation, maintenance, and suppression. Fertil Steril 33:649, 1980.
78. Jenkins S, Olive DL, Haney AF: Endometriosis: pathogenetic implications of the anatomic distribution. Obstet Gynecol 67:335, 1986.
79. Haydon GB: A study of 569 cases of endometriosis. Am J Obstet Gynecol 43:704, 1941.
80. Ranney B: Endometriosis III. Complete operations: reasons, sequelae, treatment. Am J Obstet Gynecol 109, 1137, 1971.
81. Fortier KJ, Haney AF: The pathologic spectrum of uterotubal junction obstruction. Obstet Gynecol 65:93, 1985.
82. Bates JS, Beecham CT: Retroperitoneal endometriosis with ureteral obstruction. Obstet Gynecol 34:242, 1969.
83. Roddick JW, Conkey G, Jacobs EJ: The hormonal response of endometriotic implants and its relationship to symptomatology. Am J Obstet Gynecol 79:1173, 1960.
84. Ferenczy A: Studies on the cytodynamics of human endometrial regeneration. I. Scanning electron microscopy. Am J Obstet Gynecol 124:64, 1976.
85. Frenczy A: Studies on the cytodynamics of human endometrial regeneration. II. Transmission electron microscopy and histochemistry. Am J Obstet Gynecol 124:582, 1976.
86. Lox CD, Word L, Heine MW, et al.: Ultrastructural evaluation of endometriosis. Fertil Steril 41:755, 1984.
87. Brosens I, Vasquez G, Gordts S: Scanning electron microscopic study of the pelvic peritoneum in unexplained infertility and endometriosis. Fertil Steril 41:215, 1984.
88. Prakash S, Uldelder H, Cohen RB: Enzyme-histochemical observations on endometriosis. Am J Obstet Gynecol 91:990, 1965.
89. Moon YS, Leung PCS, Yuen BH, et al.: Prostaglandin F in human endometriotic tissue. Am J Obstet Gynecol 141:344, 1981.
90. Meldrum D, Shamonki I, Clark K: Prostaglandin content of ascitic fluid in endometriosis: a preliminary report. Presented at the twenty-fifth annual meeting of the Pacific Coast Fertility Society, Palm Springs, CA: Abst 17, 1977.
91. Drake TS, O'Brien WF, Ramwell PW, et al.: Peritoneal fluid thromboxane B2 and 6-keto-prostaglandin Fla in endometriosis. Am J Obstet Gynecol 140:401, 1981.
92. Soundheimer SJ, Flickinger G: Prostaglandin F2a in the peritoneal fluid of patients with endometriosis. Int J Fertil 27:73, 1982.
93. Badawy SZA, Marshall L, Gabal AA, et al.: The concentration of 13.14-dihydro-15-keto-prostaglandin F2a and prostaglandin E2 in peritoneal fluid of infertile patients with and without endometriosis. Fertil Steril 38:166, 1982.
94. Ylikorkala O, Koskimies A, Laatkainen T, et al.: Peritoneal fluid prostaglandins in endometriosis, tubal disorders, and unexplained infertility. Obstet Gynecol 63:616, 1984.
95. Badawy SZA, Cuenca V, Marshall L, Mumchback R, Rinas AC, Coble DA: Cellular components in peritoneal fluid in infertile patients with and without endometriosis. Fertil Steril 42:704, 1984.
96. Deleon FD, Vijayakumar R, Brown M, Rao CHV, Yussman MA, Schultz G: Peritoneal fluid volume, estrogen, progesterone, prostaglandin, and epidermal growth factor concentrations in patients with and without endometriosis. Obstet Gynecol 68:189, 1986.

97. Rock JA, Dubin NH, Ghodgaonkar RB, et al: Cul-de-sac fluid in women with endometriosis: fluid volume and prostanoid concentration during the proliferative phase of the cycle - days 8 to 12. Fertil Steril 37:747, 1982.
98. Sqarlata CS, Hertelendy F, Mikhail G: The prostanoid content in peritoneal fliud and plasma of women with endometriosis. Am J Obstet Gynecol 147:563, 1983.
99. Dawood MY, Kahn-Dawood FS, Wilson L Jr: Peritoneal fluid prostaglandins and prostanoids in women with endometriosis, chronic pelvic inflammatory disease, and pelvic pain. Am J Obstet Gynecol 148:391, 1984.
100. Chacho KJ, Chaco S, Audresen PJ, Scommegma A: Peritoneal fluid in patients with and without endometriosis: prostanoids and macrophages and their effect on the spermatozoa penetration assay. Am J Obstet Gynecol 154:1290, 1986.
101. Haney AF, Handwerger S, Weinberg JB: Peritoneal fluid prolactin in infertile women with endometriosis: lack of evidence of secretory activity by endometriotic implants. Fertil Steril 42:935, 1984.
102. Janne O, Kauppila A, Kokko E, et al.: Estrogen and progestin receptors in endometriosis lesions: comparison with endometrial tissue. Am J Obstet Gynecol 141:562, 1981.
103. Bergquist A, Rannevik G, Thorell J: Estrogen and progesterone cytosol receptor concentration in endometriotic tissue and intrauterine endometrium. Acta Obstet Gynecol Scand Suppl 101:53, 1981.
104. Tamaya T, Motoyaha T, Ohono Y, et al.: Steroid receptor levels and histology of endometriosis and adenomyosis. Fertil Steril 31:396, 1979.
105. Gould SF, Shannon JM, Cunha GR: Nuclear estrogen binding sites in human endometriosis. Fertil Steril 39:520, 1983.
106. Brosens IA, Koninckx PR, Corveleyn PA: A study of plasma progesterone, oestradiol-17B, prolactin and LH levels, and of the luteal phase appearance of the ovaries in patients with endometriosis and infertility. Br J Obstet Gynecol 85:246, 1978.
107. Drake TS, Metz S, Grumert GM, O'Brien WF: Peritoneal fluid volume in endometriosis. Fertil Steril 34:280, 1980.
108. Haney AF, Muscato JJ, Weinberg JB: Peritoneal fluid cell populations in infertility patients. Fertil Steril 35:696, 1981.
109. Brews A: Endometriosis including endometriosis of the diaphragm and Meigs' syndrome. Proc R Soc Med 47:461, 1954.
110. Chervenak FA, Greenlee RM, Lewenstein L, Tovell HMM: Massive ascites associated with endometriosis. Obstet Gynecol 57:379, 1981.
111. Jenks JE, Artman LE, Hoskins WJ, Miremandi AK: Endometriosis with ascites. Obstet Gynecol 63:72s, 1984.
112. Halme J, Chafe W, Currie JL: Endometriosis with ascites. Obstet Gynecol 65:591, 1985.
113. Haney AF, Misukonis MA, Weinberg JB: Macrophages and infertility: oviductal macrophages as potential mediators of infertility. Fertil Steril 39:310, 1983.
114. Weinberg JB, Haney AF: Spontaneous tumor cell killing by human blood monocytes and peritoneal macrophages: lack of alteration by endotoxin or quenchers of oxygen species. J Natl Ca Instit 70:1005, 1983.
115. Kurlander RT, Haney AF, Gartrell J: Human peritoneal macrophages possess two populations of IgG Fc-receptors. Cell Immunol 86:479, 1984.
116. London SN, Haney AF, Weinberg JB: Macrophages and infertility: enhancement of human macrophage-mediated sperm killing by antisperm antibodies. Fertil Steril 43:274, 1985.

117. Halme J, Becker S, Hammond MG, Raj MHG, Raj S: Increased activation of pelvic macrophages in infertile women with mild endometriosis. Am J Obstet Gynecol 145:333, 1983.
118. Gleicher N, Dmowski WP, Siegel I, Liv TL, Friberg J, Radwanska E, Toder V: Lymphocyte subsets in endometriosis. Obstet Gynecol 63:463, 1984.
119. Batzofin JH, Holmes SD, Gibbons WE, Buttram VC Jr: Peritoneal fluid plasminogen activator activity in endometriosis and pelvic adhesive disease. Fertil Steril 44:277, 1985.
120. Weed JC, Arquembourg PC, Endometriosis: can it produce an autoimmune response resulting in infertility? Clinical Obstet Gynecol 23:885, 1980.
121. Bartosik D, Viscarello RR, Damjanov I: Endometriosis as an autoimmune disease. Fertil Steril 41:215, 1984.
122. Badway SZA, Guenca V, Stitzel A, Jacobs RDB, Tomar RH: Autoimmune phenomena in infertile patients with endometriosis. Obstet Gynecol 63:271, 1984.
123. Mathur S, Peress MR, Williamson HO, Youmans CD, Maney SA, Garvin AJ, Rust PF, Fudenberg HH: Autoimmunity to endometrium and ovary in endometriosis. Clin Exp Immunol 50:259, 1982.
124. Steele RW, Dmowski WP, Marmar DJ: Immunologic aspects of human endometriosis. Am J Reprod Immunol 6:33, 1984.
125. Halme J, Becker S, Haskill S: Altered lifespan and function of peritoneal macrophages: a new hypothesis for pathogenesis of endometriosis. Presented at the thirty-third annual meeting of the Society for Gynecologic Investigation, Toronto, Abst 48, 1986.
126. Kabawat SE, Bast RC Jr, Bhan AK, Welch WR, Knapp RC, Colvin RB: Tissue distribution of a coelomic-epithelium-related antigen recognized by the monoclonal antibody OC-125. Int J Gynecol Pathol 2:275, 1983.
127. Bast RC Jr, Klug TL, St. John E, Jenisom E, Niloff JM, Lazarus H, Berkowitz RS, Leavitt T, Griffiths CT, Parker L, Zurawski VR Jr, Knapp RC: A radioimmunoassay using a monoclonal antibody to monitor the course of epithelial ovarian cancer. N Engl J Med 309:883, 1983.
128. Niloff JM, Knapp RC, Schaetzl E, Reynolds C, Bast RC Jr: CA-125 antigen levels in obstetric and gynecologic patients. Obstet Gynecol 64:703, 1984.
129. Barbieri RL, Niloff JM, Bast RC Jr, Schaetzl E, Kistner RW, Knapp RC: Elevated serum concentrations of CA-125 in patients with advanced endometriosis. Fertil Steril 45:630, 1986.
130. Guidice LC, Jacobs A, Pineda J, Bell CE, Lippmann L: Serum levels of CA-125 in patients with endometriosis. Fertil Steril 45:876, 1986.
131. Patton PE, Field CS, Harms RW, Coulam CB: CA-125 levels in endometriosis. Fertil Steril 45:770, 1986.

Endometriosis, pages 53–77

Chapter 4
Clinical Presentation and Diagnosis

Robert A. Wild, M.D., and Emery A. Wilson, M.D.

Hershey Medical Center, Pennsylvania State University, Hershey, Pennsylvania 17033 (R.A.W.) and Division of Reproductive Endocrinology, Kentucky Center for Reproductive Medicine, Lexington, Kentucky 40536 (E.A.W.)

INTRODUCTION

The characteristic symptoms and signs of endometriosis readily lead to its diagnosis, but the clinical presentation of this enigmatic disorder is not always characteristic. The symptoms may be highly variable from one patient to another, and the magnitude of symptoms may not correlate with the extent of the disease. For example, patients with mild endometriosis may have incapacitating pain, whereas patients with severe disease can be asymptomatic. The likelihood of infertility does tend to increase as the severity of disease increases, but the diagnosis of endometriosis, particularly the milder forms, is still often delayed.

The purpose of this chapter is to enhance awareness of the common symptoms and signs of this disorder. Increasing physician awareness of endometriosis and its effects is probably the first step toward diagnosis, which must be confirmed by direct visualization. Milder forms of endometriosis may present in a subtle manner even under direct visualization, and the clinician should have not only a knowledge of endometriosis and surgical experience locating it but should also be aware of certain pitfalls in the diagnosis of this disorder. Current diagnostic research focuses on laboratory techniques that would prompt clinicians to consider endometriosis earlier in the evaluation of a patient's complaints.

SITES OF ENDOMETRIOSIS OCCURRENCE

The clinical presentation and symptoms of endometriosis frequently relate to the anatomical location of the disease. Although endometriosis can be present at distant sites (see Chapter 11), it is usually confined to the pelvis. In a study mapping the composite findings in 516 patients, Scott et al. [1] tabulated the sites of endometriosis implants (Fig. 1). All patients had histologically verified lesions. The most common sites of involvement were the ovaries, pelvic peritoneum, cul-de-sac, uterosacral ligaments, and posterior uterine surface. Assuming that endometriosis occurs as a result of retrograde menstruation through the oviducts, the erect position of the human

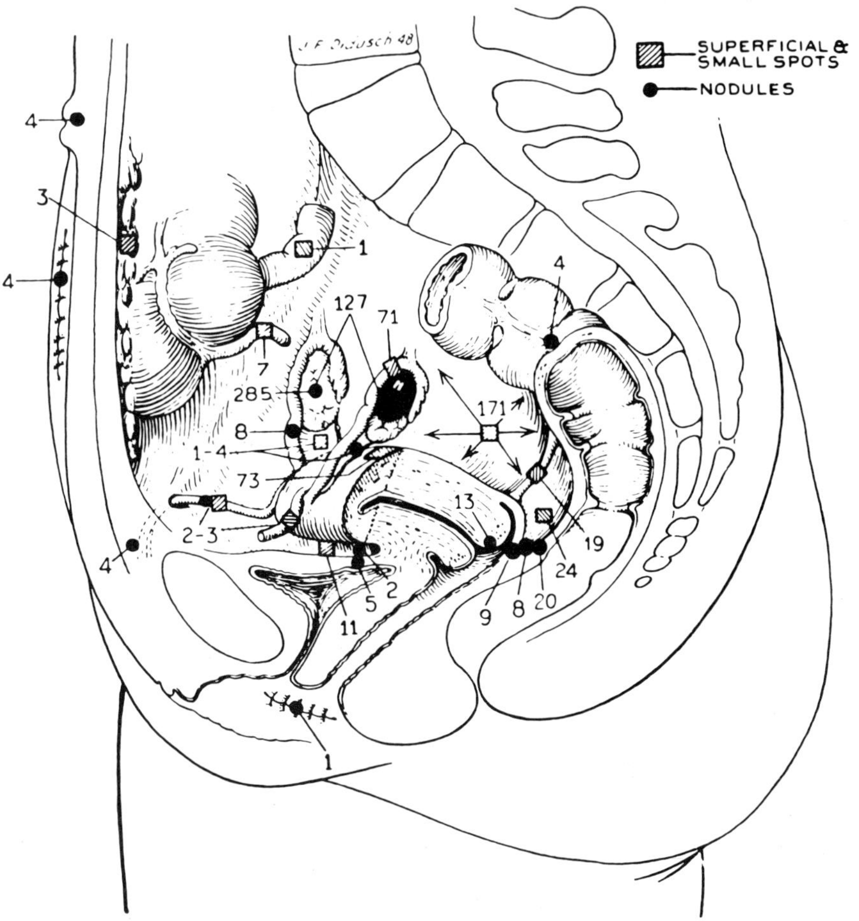

Fig. 1. Location of external endometriosis in 516 cases. The numbers add to more than 516 because of multiple types and locations of lesions in single cases. Reprinted with permission: Scott et al. External endometriosis: the scourge of the private patient. Ann Surg 131: 706, 1950.

female predisposes to the collection of endometrial tissue in these areas. The next most common sites were the serosal surfaces of the rectosigmoid colon, bladder, ileum, appendix, and round ligaments. In a series of patients with both infertility and endometriosis diagnosed by laparoscopy, Jenkins et al. [2] found a similar distribution of lesions and offered the data to support retrograde menstruation as the primary mode of development (see Chapter 3).

CLINICAL OBSERVATIONS

The following clinical observations in patients with endometriosis are pertinent to the clinical presentation: 1) endometriosis is a disease of women during reproductive age, 2) the disease occurs only after menarche, 3) with rare exceptions [3–5] it is of no serious consequence after menopause except as it is related to ovarian cancer, 4) it is common in women who have uninterrupted cyclic menstruation for periods exceeding 5 years, 5) it seems to be encountered less commonly in women with anovulatory cycles, 6) endometriosis improves both subjectively and objectively during periods of physiologically induced (pregnancy) and artificially induced anovulation (danazol therapy), 7) frequent pregnancies, if initiated early in menstrual life, seem to prevent, at least temporarily, development of the disorder, 8) endometriosis is commonly associated with infertility, and 9) the disease seems to occur in families.

CLINICAL PATHOLOGICAL CORRELATION

The most common site of endometriosis is the ovary, and in about one-half of the cases both ovaries are involved. In its early development, it may occur either as small, bluish, punctate hemorrhagic areas on the surface of the ovary or as small cysts lying beneath the surface epithelium. During early stages of development, cysts become adherent to surrounding structures, particularly the broad ligament and the serosa of the sigmoid colon. A typical picture of ovarian endometriosis is illustrated in Figure 2.

Usually the tubes are patent and not involved in early endometriosis. Not uncommonly a convoluted and edematous oviduct is observed. With progression of the disease, the distal oviduct can become adherent to the ovary, resulting in diminished motility and presumably inadequate ovum pick up.

Benign endometrial ovarian cysts may vary from microscopic to 8–10 cm in diameter (Fig. 3). Large endometrial cysts measuring 15 cm in diameter are not unheard of in reproductive-age women who are symptomatic. Endo-

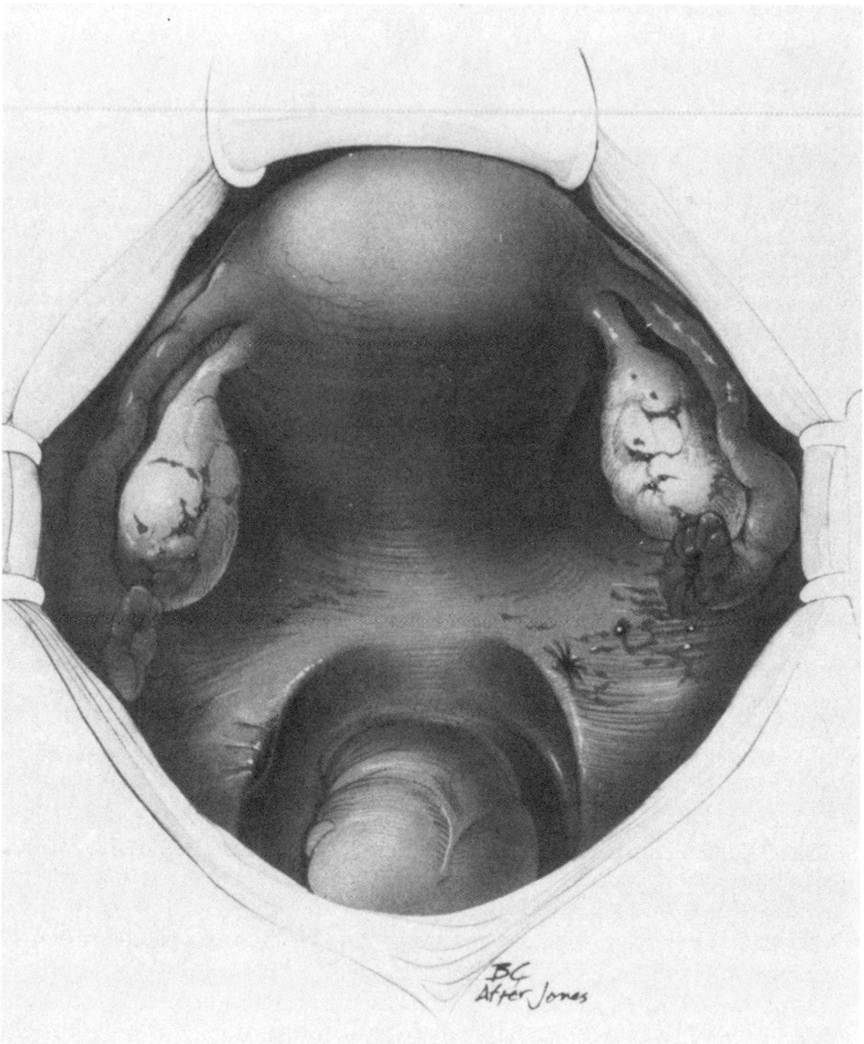

Fig. 2. Early endometriosis involving the peritoneum and ovary. From: A.H. Curtis Textbook of Gynecology, ed. 5. Philadelphia: W.B. Saunders Co., 1946, p. 547.

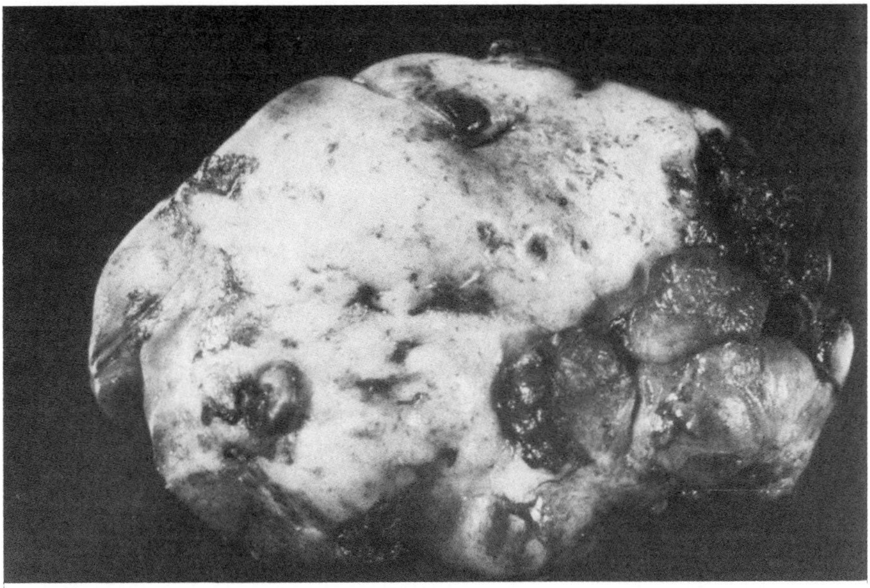

Fig. 3. Ovarian endometrioma (Courtesy of Richard Zaino, M.D., Dept. of Pathology, Hershey Medical Center, Pennsylvania State University, Hershey, PA).

metrial cysts may be multiple in early stages, but subsequently coalesce into a single large cyst (Fig. 4). The lining of an endometrial ovarian cyst varies from red to dark brown, depending on the extent and duration of bleeding. Depending on the amount of functioning endometrium, it may be thick and velvety or thin and smooth (Fig. 5). Continuing function in endometriosis implants tends to destroy its microscopic characteristics and, thus, follows Dr. Arthur Hertig's observation many years ago, "The more advanced the lesion clinically, the poorer the histological detail [6]"

Small areas of surface endometriosis tend to rupture rather early in development. This can produce adhesions, pelvic dissemination, and pain. Deeper areas tend to grow slowly and gradually enlarge as intracystic bleeding occurs. The capsule becomes thickened. Therefore, spontaneous rupture of large endometriomas, which can cause chemical peritonitis in a previously asymptomatic woman, is rare.

There are four basic microscopic elements seen with endometriosis: 1) endometrial epithelium, 2) glands or glandlike structures, 3) stroma, and 4) hemorrhage (Fig. 6). Early lesions usually demonstrate classic histology, whereas a large endometrioma obvious at the operating table may have only hemosiderin-laden macrophages, with varying amounts of fibrous connective

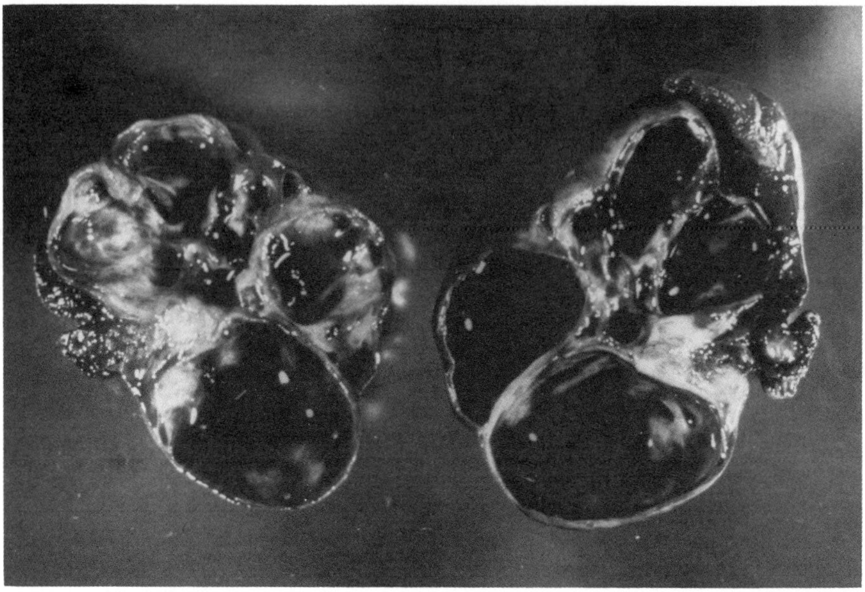

Fig. 4. Multiple endometrial cysts, subsequent coalescence (Courtesy of Richard Zaino, M.D., Dept. of Pathology, Hershey Medical Center, Pennsylvania State University, Hershey, PA).

tissue and inflammatory cells reported. This inflammatory response may hold clues to understanding the pathophysiology of the disorder (Chapter 3).

It is important to remember that the stroma, not the glands or epithelium, is responsible for bleeding in endometriosis. The diagnosis of endometriosis can be suspected by an experienced gynecologic pathologist by the presence of stroma alone.

SYMPTOMS

The symptoms characteristic for endometriosis include: 1) progressive acquired pelvic pain associated with or occurring just prior to menstruation, 2) dyspareunia, 3) painful defecation, 4) premenstrual staining and abnormal bleeding, 5) suprapubic pain, dysuria, and hematuria, and 6) infertility.

The clinical diagnosis of endometriosis is based on the characteristic symptoms and physical findings. However, the symptoms may be highly variable. A patient with extensive endometriosis may be incapacitated with pain or may be totally asymptomatic. The same variability of symptoms exists, for the patient with mild endometriosis. In a study of 513 patients with

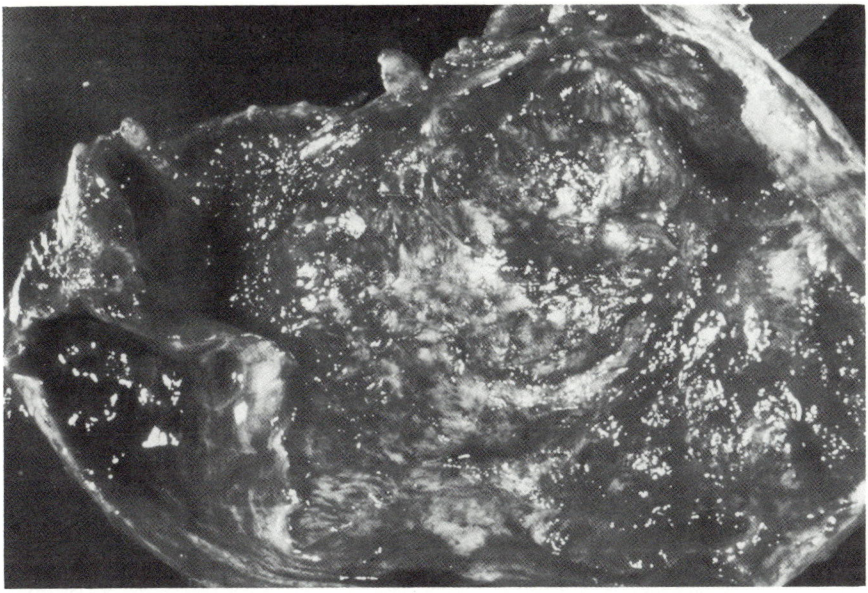

Fig. 5. Inner wall of an ovarian endometrioma (Courtesy of Richard Zaino, M.D., Dept. of Pathology, Hershey Medical Center, Pennsylvania State University, Hershey, PA).

infertility and endometriosis confirmed at laparoscopy, Cohen reported that 64% of these patients were asymptomatic [7]. Therefore, if the classical symptoms and physical findings are present, the diagnosis can be straightforward, but the absence of symptoms and physical findings does not mean that endometriosis is not present.

Pain

Pelvic pain, dysmenorrhea in particular, is a cardinal symptom of patients with endometriosis. Some patients state that they always have had painful periods. Most will, however, admit to a recent increase in severity. The pain is usually lateral, not suprapubic. Often, it is described as being "deep inside," constant, and frequently referred to the rectal area. As the disease progresses, the pain may be present throughout the month, not just at the time of menses.

The cause of the pain has not been well defined. It is speculated that it is related to miniature menstruation and bleeding in areas that are totally or partially encapsulated by fibrous tissue or peritoneum. Cyclic swelling and bleeding within the implants may stretch surrounding tissues. Another con-

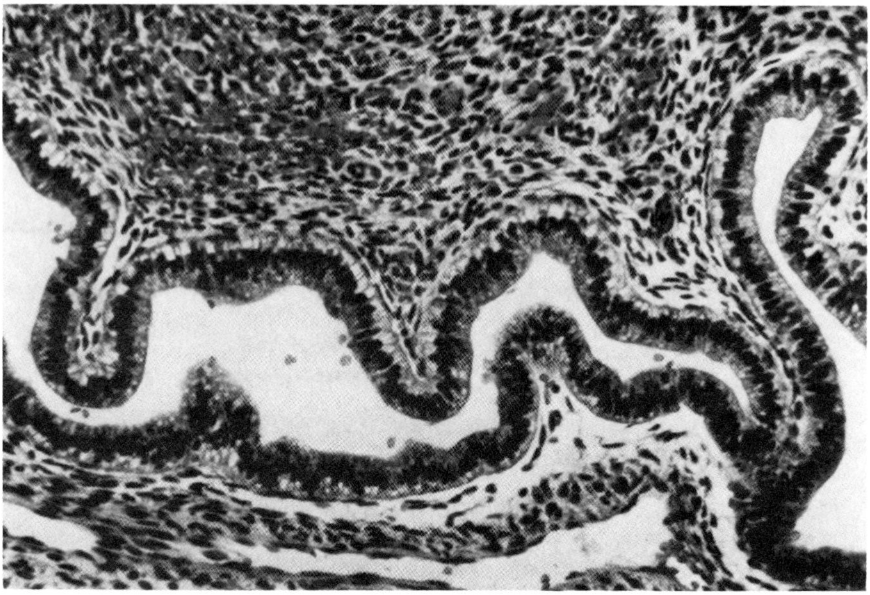

Fig. 6. Microscopic appearance of endometriosis with elements 1) endometrial epithelium; 2) glands or glandlike structures; 3) stroma; 4) hemorrhage (Courtesy of Richard Zaino, M.D., Dept. of Pathology, Hershey Medical Center, Pennsylvania State University, Hershey, PA).

tributing factor may be the production of prostaglandins within the ectopic endometrium [8] (see Chapter 3). A number of these compounds are potent mediators of inflammation. Prostaglandins also may sensitize nerve endings to pain stimuli [9]. Early in the disease process, the late luteal and early menstrual phases are when prostaglandin release from in situ endometrium markedly increases [10]. On the other hand, the lack of consistent relief of endometriosis-related pain by prostaglandin synthetase inhibitors [11] would suggest that local mechanical factors predominate. Pain is not always associated with endometriosis, even when the disease is extensive. Bilateral, large ovarian endometriomas develop slowly and frequently are asymptomatic unless rupture occurs, whereas incapacitating pelvic discomfort may be associated with minimal amounts of active endometriosis. The tendency toward an inverse relationship between the amount of disease and the amount of pain has led to the suggestion that extensive disease may eventually destroy nerve endings.

Dyspareunia is a common symptom, particularly with deep penetration, and may play a role in any associated infertility. Functioning endometriosis in the posterior cul-de-sac, causing fixed uterine retroversion, is a ready explanation. Why some women may have severe dysmenorrhea and others with the same extent of disease can be totally asymptomatic is not fully understood.

Pain and other symptoms can also be experienced when endometriosis involves other organ systems. The presence of endometriosis implants on the rectum and sigmoid colon results in bleeding into the muscularis or serosa and often causes pain with defecation. For many patients, these symptoms are expressed as rectal pressure or an urgency to defecate, particularly during menses. Bloody stools may occur during the premenstrual or menstrual phases. With increasing encroachment of endometriosis on the bowel wall, crampy pain typical of partial bowel obstruction may be experienced.

Suprapubic, bearing down discomfort at the time of menstruation may be associated with dysuria and hematuria due to the extension of the disease into the muscularis of the bladder. Abdominal and flank pain can occur because of ureteral obstruction with development of hydroureter and hydronephrosis. Urinary tract endometriosis is uncommon, but probably occurs more frequently than reported in the literature. The pelvic ureter more frequently is involved than is deep invasion of the bladder (Fig. 7). Endometriosis of the serosal surfaces of the bladder, although extremely common, is usually asymptomatic. By the time the muscularis or mucosa is involved, patients usually have noted cyclic hematuria and pain. The areas of involvement are usually in the dome of the bladder. The trigone is rarely involved. If it is, it usually is secondary to extensive vaginal and/or cervical involvement by endometriosis. Ureteral involvement has been reported with increasing frequency [12–15] and probably explains many cases of idiopathic cyclic unilateral hydronephrosis. Flank pain and fever during premenstrual and menstrual phases of the cycle may be a clue. Pyuria and hematuria may occur from intermittent ureteral obstruction.

Endometriosis at distant sites such as the lung or pleura can result in symptoms specific to that organ system. For example, endometriosis in the lung can cause catamenial pneumothorax or hemoptysis. The symptoms and management of endometriosis effects on other organ systems are discussed in Chapter 11.

Endometriosis can always coexist with other disorders that may in part be responsible for the patient's symptoms. Egger and Weigmann [16] reviewed the case histories of 263 patients with histologically proven endometriotic ovarian cysts and found that 42% of patients had uterine leiomyomas and 42% also had adenomyosis. There were 48 other unrelated major diagnoses such as cancer of the cervix or endometrium in this group of patients. However, the risk of carcinoma in endometriosis was less than 1%.

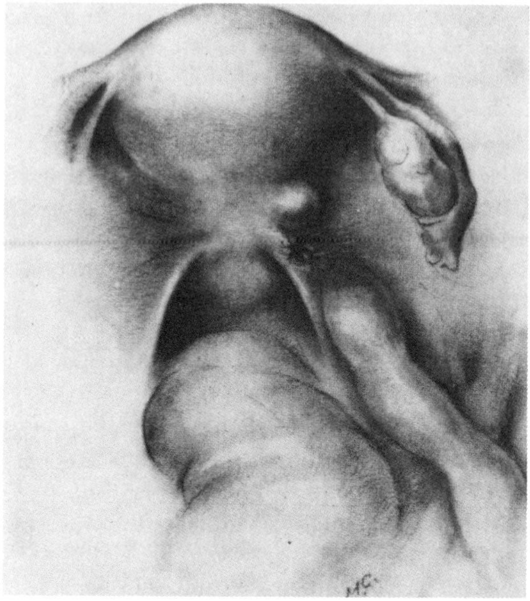

Fig. 7. Endometriosis involving the right uterosacral ligament, with fibrosis producing marked right hydroureter. (Reproduced with permission from Kistner, R.W.: "Gynecology: Principles and Practice." 4th edition. 1986. Chicago: Year Book Medical Publishers, Inc.)

The pain associated with endometriosis may be acute or chronic, and although it is usually restricted to the perimenstrual period, pain may actually occur throughout the cycle. In addition to endometriosis implants, patients may also have associated pelvic adhesions or endometriomas of the ovaries as a source of pelvic pain. In patients undergoing diagnostic laparoscopy to confirm the presence of endometriosis, 32–41% of patients experienced chronic pain [17–18]. When ovarian endometriotic cysts are present, lower abdominal pain has been reported to be present in as many as 72% of patients [16].

At times, the use of medications can be helpful in the diagnosis of endometriosis and in distinguishing it from other disorders. Antiprostaglandin agents and oral contraceptives are helpful in relieving primary dysmenorrhea and painful ovulation, but even patients with endometriosis may benefit some from these agents. Medications that are specifically used for the treatment of endometriosis, such as danazol, may also relieve pelvic pain, but the clinician should not assume a diagnosis of endometriosis without direct visualization or biopsy.

Menstrual Characteristics and Bleeding Abnormalities

There is a trend for women with endometriosis to have an earlier menarche than other women (see Chapter 2). Cramer and associates [19] have reported that women with endometriosis tend to have an earlier menarche, shorter menstrual cycles, and a longer duration of menses than other women. However, Wilson and colleagues [20] found that women with endometriosis reported a significant decrease in menstrual duration and decrease in menstrual flow when patients compare their present menstrual characteristics to menstrual characteristics several years previously. Part of this discrepancy may be explained by the amount of intermenstrual spotting in endometriosis patients. Intermenstrual spotting is actually more common in all groups of infertility patients than in fertile patients [20] and, thus, metrorrhagia may be more associated with infertility than endometriosis alone.

Premenstrual spotting may occur in patients with endometriosis. Although premenstrual spotting has long been thought to be due to inadequate luteal phase progesterone production, Wentz [21] found that this symptom is observed commonly in patients with endometriosis and that it is rare in patients with luteal phase inadequacy.

Infertility

The incidence of infertility in patients with endometriosis has been reported to be as high as 66% [22], and 25% to 35% of patients undergoing laparoscopy for infertility can be found to have endometriosis [18]. The relationship between endometriosis and infertility is covered more extensively in Chapter 6, but the diagnosis of endometriosis should always be considered in patients with infertility. In fact, the association is so common that if no obvious cause of infertility is determined with infertility screening studies or if the patient does not respond readily to appropriate therapy for infertility, a diagnostic laparoscopy should be performed in search of endometriosis.

Although the association between infertility and endometriosis will be covered more extensively later, certain symptoms relating to infertility may be important for the diagnosis of endometriosis. In this regard, patients with endometriosis have been reported to be more likely to have anovulation with irregular menses, luteal phase defects that may result in shorter menstrual cycles, and hyperprolactinemia that may cause galactorrhea [23]. In any patient with infertility who has one or more of these associated symptoms, endometriosis should be considered.

Spontaneous Abortion

Several investigators [24–27] have suggested an increased incidence of spontaneous abortion in patients with endometriosis, with a return to normal abortion rate after medical or surgical treatment. While the link between autoimmune factors and spontaneous abortion with endometriosis is theoretically very attractive and certainly remains to be explored, a major criticism of studies showing increased rate of pregnancy wastage contributed to endometriosis is a lack of a control group derived from the patient population being studied. Metzger et al. [28] recently called attention to this problem comparing 139 consecutive fertility patients with laparoscopically proven endometriosis to determine the incidence of spontaneous abortion. "Expectant management" was found to have a reduction in spontaneous abortion rate as well. They suggested that the spontaneous abortion rate in untreated endometriosis may not be as high as previously reported and may not be significantly different from the rate in the general population. While major problems exist in designing the appropriate control group for evaluation, this problem, like so many others attempting to study endometriosis, reflects the hazards of bias of ascertainment and lack of prospective randomized study designs with adequate numbers of patients to offer definitive conclusions.

Family History

The classic symptoms addressed above may or may not be present in the patient's history. A history of infertility is common. A family history of infertility, endometriosis, or hysterectomy can often be elicited. While familial tendencies have been observed and reported consistently [29,30], systematic pedigree analyses were performed by Simpson et al. on the relatives of 123 patients with endometriosis [31] and, as controls, the relatives of the patients' husbands. First-degree relatives of patients had a 6.9% occurrence of endometriosis as compared with 1% overall occurrence in the husbands' female relatives. This gives us minimal estimates of the presence of endometriosis in relatives and a basis for patient counseling. The figure suggests there is some inherent factor conferring increased susceptibility to the development of this disorder. Theories of pathogenesis must take into account this recognized familial tendency.

PHYSICAL DIAGNOSIS

The physical examination is helpful in discerning if endometriosis may be present. However, other disorders can cause the same findings on examination and none of these findings are specific for endometriosis.

Cul-de-sac Tenderness and Nodularity

Classically, pelvic examination reveals tender nodules present in the posterior vaginal fornix and along the uterosacral ligaments. Endometriosis nodules may be exquisitely tender to palpitation and may be best palpated on rectal-vaginal examination.

Adnexal Mass

The ovary is the most common site for endometriosis, which may be manifested as an endometrioma or an adnexal mass caused by periovarian adhesions. As stated previously, ovarian endometriosis may also coexist with uterine leiomyomas or other disorders presenting as an adnexal mass.

Endometriosis should be suspected if a patient of reproductive age presents with an adnexal mass or if the patient with infertility can be shown to have a persistent adnexal mass or ovarian enlargement. One-third of the patients who present with endometriomas have bilateral endometriotic cysts [16]. Certainly any persistent ovarian cyst should be investigated surgically. Although the risk for carcinoma in endometriotic cysts is less than 1% [16], neoplastic disorders of the ovary and adjacent tissues can easily be mistaken for endometriosis.

Uterine Retrodisplacement

Endrometriosis posterior to the uterus frequently causes obliteration of the cul-de-sac and progressive development of scar tissue pulls the uterus posteriorly into a retrodisplaced position. A fixed, retrodisplaced uterus on pelvic examination is suggestive of endometriosis, and this sign is usually associated with more advanced disease. However, a retrodisplaced uterus can be a variant of a normal pelvis and not all patients with a retrodisplaced uterus have endometriosis. Friedman and coworkers [32] found laparoscopic evidence of endometriosis in only one-third of the patients with a retrodisplaced uterus.

Other Physical Findings

Endometriosis can be detected in episiotomies, vaginal lacerations, abdominal wall incisions, or occasionally other areas that can be detected on physical examination. The presence of dark blue or brown nodules in these areas should suggest endometriosis, particularly if they become more tender and increase in size during menses.

Patients who have previously had a hysterectomy for endometriosis or other disorders may have implants of endometriosis at the apex of the vaginal vault. In the presence of continued hormonal stimulation, either by ovaries left in place or by exogenous hormones, endometriosis can cause cyclic bleeding. Thus, persistent cyclic bleeding in a patient who has previously undergone hysterectomy should suggest endometriosis.

DIFFERENTIAL DIAGNOSIS

The varied presentations of endometriosis mandate that it must be considered in the differential diagnosis of virtually all pelvic diseases. In particular, the pain, infertility, and adhesions associated with endometriosis should be distinguished from similar symptoms that may accompany primary or secondary dysmenorrhea, pelvic inflammatory disease, pelvic neoplasia, benign or malignant ovarian lesions, uterine leiomyomas, gastrointestinal pathology, and urological pathology. Usually, differentiation between endometriosis and these other disorders requires operative evaluation.

Uterine Adenomyosis

Also known as internal endometriosis, adenomyosis is the invasion and growth of normal endometrium into the myometrium. It is usually characterized by a clinical presentation quite different from that of endometriosis. In certain conditions, however, symptoms can be quite similar in that pelvic pain, hypermenorrhea, and intermenstrual staining are common to both processes. Adenomyosis usually occurs in older, gravid women, approximately age 35–50. Pelvic pain and hypermenorrhea in a woman who has had several children and for whom infertility has not been a problem is the classic story. The adenomyotic uterus is usually symmetrically enlarged and tender. The cul-de-sac and ovaries are not involved.

Ovarian Pathology

Bleeding from a corpus luteum or a follicular cyst may be asymptomatic but, in certain cases, may be confused with endometriosis. Furthermore, every chocolate cyst of the ovary is not caused by endometriosis, because hemorrhagic follicular and corpus luteum cysts may produce a similar gross appearance. A patient with a persistent adnexal mass greater than 5 cm should never be presumed to have an endometrioma, even if endometriosis has been diagnosed previously.

Malignancy in endometriosis is rare (less than 1%) and usually presents as a well-differentiated adenocarcinoma or adenocanthoma (Fig. 8). The tumors tend to be larger than the benign form of endometrioma, averaging 8 to 9 cm. The prognosis is considerably better than that associated with ovarian cancer in general. It is possible, of course, that many ovarian cancers originate in endometriosis, but are so undifferentiated when discovered that precise determination of origin is impossible. Criteria for the diagnosis of carcinoma arising in endometriosis are: 1) the involved ovary must be the site of endometriosis, 2) there must be a genuine adenocarcinoma, 3) a transition from benign to malignant areas must be demonstrated, 4) the

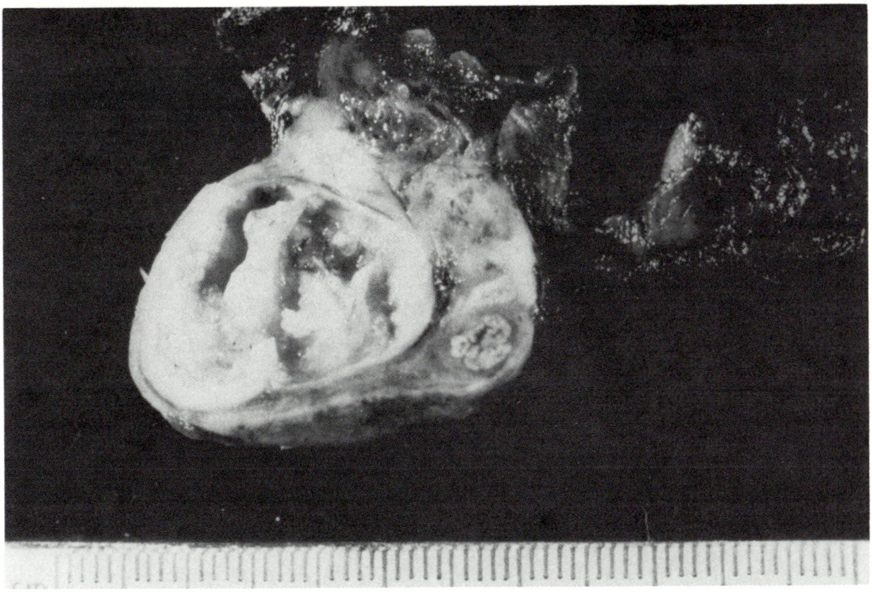

Fig. 8. Low-grade malignancy arising in an ovarian endometrioma (Courtesy of Richard Zaino, M.D., Dept. of Pathology, Hershey Medical Center, Pennsylvania State University, Hershey, PA).

endometrium must not show adenocarcinoma. These tumors are prone to local invasion but metastasize rarely. Although the likelihood of carcinoma is rare in a patient suspected of having endometriosis, malignancies certainly can occur in women during the reproductive years. The clinician must be aware of the possibilities of malignancy during the preoperative evaluation.

Pelvic Inflammatory Disease

Chronic pelvic inflammatory disease with bilateral adherent adnexal masses, because of its variable clinical presentation and the frequency of its occurrence, is the condition most frequently confused with endometriosis. An infected ovarian cyst may present with the same clinical picture as a pelvic or tubo-ovarian abscess and is diagnosed rarely prior to surgery. With pelvic inflammatory disease, pelvic examination often reveals tender, bilateral broad ligament masses that have a characteristic fluctuant and doughy consistency. Fever is usually present. Objective and subjective improvement usually follows appropriate antibiotic therapy if rupture of the abscess has not occurred. Laparoscopic examination may be necessary for diagnosis. Unilateral acute pyosalpinx has been recognized with increasing frequency.

Rupture of an ovarian endometrioma may simulate appendicitis, ectopic pregnancy, pelvic peritonitis, twisted adnexa, rupture of an ovarian follicle hematoma, or almost any acute pelvic process.

Endometriosis can lead to hematosalpinx. This rather unusual process must be differentiated from an ectopic pregnancy. Sensitive hCG testing has aided greatly in differentiating this disorder. An hematosalpinx caused by endometriosis may occur in a tube previously damaged by pelvic infection. Just as endosalpingiosis of the cornua develops in or near the transition from endometrium to tubal epithelium, endometriosis can develop at the mucosa-serosal junction on the fimbriated end of the oviduct. It is also possible for endometriosis to occur in other parts of the oviduct, particularly the ampulla. If the fimbria becomes sealed, the endometriosis may cause an hematosalpinx.

The condition of nodular thickening of the proximal oviducts, referred to as salpingitis isthmica nodosa, is characterized more by speculation than accumulation of factual knowledge concerning its etiology, incidence, and clinical significance. Controversy still prevails as to whether the origin of salpingitis isthmica nodosa is postinflammatory, congenital, or acquired (analogous to adenomyosis of the uterus) [33]. It is associated with tubal pregnancy [33] and has a characteristic radiological appearance [34]. From the standpoint of pathogenesis, the condition seems to be caused by mucosal alteration starting from the luminal surface of the oviducts and extending into the muscularis. The term endosalpingoblastosis has been proposed as a more descriptive term [33]. Two types are suggested depending on whether the glandular component is tubal or endometrial in origin.

Endometriosis of the oviduct is histologically distinct from and should not be confused with salpingitis isthmica nodosa. Radiologically the honeycombed tubal appearance in the proximal segment of the oviduct due to endometriosis appears as thicker diverticulae associated with a normal uterus and patent tubes [35]. One interesting report noted a 74% patency rate (42.8% pregnancy rate) after high-dose progestin therapy in 112 patients with uterotubal junction obstruction of unknown etiology [36]. Presumably, many of these patients had endometriosis of the tube. Salat-Baroux and colleagues noted endometriosis to be the cause of obstruction in 34 of 48 patients with isthmic tubal obstruction [37].

Disorders of the Urological and Gastrointestinal Tracts

Hematuria or rectal bleeding at the time of menses is highly indicative of perforating endometriosis of the bladder or rectosigmoid colon, but intrinsic disease of the bladder and colon should be investigated. Cystoscopy and sigmoidscopy may facilitate diagnosis, and biopsy is occasionally necessary.

Upper and lower GI roentgenography as well as colonoscopy are at times very useful. Endometriosis can mimic the presentation of Crohn's disease or cancer of the bowel, with extreme difficulty in differential diagnosis. In general, endometriosis invades the bowel from the serosal surface, and, therefore, the lesion is extrinsic to the bowel lumen in contrast to colon cancer, which originates in the mucosa.

DIAGNOSIS

History suggests endometriosis, pelvic examination corroborates it, and direct visualization or biopsy verifies it. The definitive diagnosis of endometriosis can only be made by direct observation of endometriosis implants at endoscopy or laparotomy. Laparoscopy has essentially replaced culdoscopy as the preferred endoscopic method because visualization of pelvic organs is better and operative techniques are easier to employ.

Laparoscopy

Laparoscopy is indicated in 1) any infertile woman in whom the infertility screening studies have been normal, 2) any couple with unexplained infertility, 3) cases of suspected endometriosis, 4) cases of abnormal hysterosalpingogram, 5) patients with suspected pelvic inflammatory disease, 6) patients suspected of having pelvic adhesions, 7) some patients to confirm ovarian dysfunction, 8) patients to evaluate the results of therapy for endometriosis or other pelvic disorders, 9) patients to evaluate accessibility of the ovaries for ovum retrieval, 10) patients undergoing ovum retrieval for gamete intrafallopian transfer (GIFT), and 11) patients undergoing ovum retrieval for subsequent in vitro fertilization and embryo transfer.

In a study to compare the incidence of unsuspected pelvic abnormalities in fertile and in infertile women at the time of diagnostic laparoscopy, Drake and Grunert [38] found endometriosis in 48% of the infertile group of patients but in only 5% of the fertile group. Seventy-nine percent of the infertile group had previously unsuspected abnormalities at the time of laparoscopy. This is an extraordinarily high rate of positive findings at laparoscopy, because other investigators report abnormalities in the 25% to 50% range, but it does emphasize the need for diagnostic laparoscopy in patients presenting with infertility, pelvic pain, and other disorders.

Contraindications to laparoscopy include medical contraindications to anesthesia, extensive adhesions from previous abdominal surgery, and disorders of infertility that cannot be otherwise treated, such as ovarian failure or absolute male infertility.

The optimal time for performing laparoscopy during the menstrual cycle depends on what abnormalities are being investigated and, to some extent, personal preference of the patient and physician. If the procedure is performed during the follicular phase of the cycle, the patient and physician are reassured that no pregnancy would be interrupted and that the endometrium had not grown to the point of obstructing the fallopian tubes, which would interfere with tubal insufflation. On the other hand, if laparoscopy is performed in the early luteal phase, valuable information can be obtained regarding ovulation. After ovulation, a frcsh hcmorrhagic corpus luteum with the stigma where ovulation has occurred can be seen. Although evaluation of the pelvis for the presence of endometriosis can be performed in either the follicular or luteal phase of the cycle, ovarian dysfunction associated with endometriosis may be best evaluated in the luteal phase. Not only can the ovaries be examined for the stigma of ovulation, but peritoneal fluid can be obtained and evaluated for volume, macrophages, steroid hormone concentrations typical of ovulation or luteinized but unruptured follicles, and other ovulatory disorders associated with endometriosis (see Chapter 6).

A systematic approach to the laparoscopic evaluation of the pelvis for endometriosis or other disorders assures that all parts of the pelvic anatomy are investigated and, if the same systematic approach is used in dictating the operative note, all pertinent information is included. For example, one approach would be to examine first the bladder, uterus, cul-de-sac, and uterosacral ligaments; then the right tube and right ovary; then the left tube and left ovary. Both tubes and ovaries should be totally accessible and freely movable. The tubes and ovaries should be elevated to assure that no endometriosis is present between the tube and ovary or between the ovary and the peritoneal surface. It is not unusual for patients with endometriosis to have adhesions that bind the ovary to the posterior peritoneal surface, so the ovary should be elevated to look for both endometriosis implants and adhesions. It is equally important to record negative information in the operative report so that other physicians can obtain as much information as possible from the report. If the tubes and ovaries are freely movable, it should be so stated. If no endometriosis is detected, the operative note should state that endometriosis was considered and that none was seen. Finally, the operative note should also indicate what percentage of the surface of each ovary is accessible for ovum retrieval should the patient ever be a candidate for in vitro fertilization and embryo transfer.

Diagnosis of endometriosis at laparascopy or laparotomy requires both a knowledge of pelvic anatomy as well as experience in the recognition of endometriosis implants and where they are likely to be found. During laparoscopy, the gross appearance of established endometriosis is usually obvious. It appears as brownish, bluish, or purplish hemorrhagic areas often associated with stellate scarring. The implants are typically found on the serosa of the bladder and posterior uterus, cul-de-sac, uterosacral ligaments, and ovaries. They may range in size from 1 to 2 mm implants to endometriomas several centimeters in diameter. Pelvic adhesions may also be present and these are often found between the tubes and ovaries and between the ovaries and the posterior peritoneal surface. Endometriosis usually does not cause obstruction of the fimbriated ends of the fallopian tubes except in patients with extensive disease. Therefore, if pelvic adhesions involve the ovaries but the fallopian tubes remain patent, endometriosis should always be considered. The uterus may be retrodisplaced and the rectum may be stuck to the posterior uterine surface, ablating the cul-de-sac.

Although the classical "burned out" lesions of endometriosis are easily identified, some of the more subtle forms of endometriosis should not be overlooked. Endometriosis may also present as white plaques, petechial lesions, eccymoses, or similar lesions associated with typical stellate scarring. Some of these subtle lesions may actually be more likely to interfere with fertility than the typical "burned out" implants [39] (see Chapter 5). Hemosiderin deposits may also be observed, and although hemosiderin is not diagnostic of endometriosis, it should suggest the presence of endometrial implants. Chatman [40] found that pelvic peritoneal defects may be associated with endometriosis. In 25 patients found to have small tears or defects in the peritoneum, 68% had associated endometriosis. Certainly, when such defects are noted at diagnostic laparoscopy, the presence of other associated pathology including endometriosis should be investigated.

A number of ancillary procedures can often be performed during a diagnostic laparoscopy for the treatment of endometriosis. Filmy adhesions can be lysed using scissors or laser techniques. Laser vaporization of endometriosis implants has been advocated by some investigators. The advantages and disadvantages of laser surgery are presented in Chapter 8. In addition, endometriosis implants can be cauterized. The pelvis can be irrigated with heparinized Ringer's lactate solution, or 32% dextron 70 (Hyskon) can be left in the peritoneal cavity to prevent development of further adhesions.

Documentation of endometriosis and the extent of pelvic disease at the time of diagnostic laparoscopy is helpful. All patients should be staged by the American Fertility Society Revised Classification (see Chapter 5). Photographs taken through the laparoscope can document the presence of endometriosis, and they can also be used to compare treatment modalities. Photographs are particularly helpful for the permanent record or when a patient is to be referred to another physician for subsequent surgery or other forms of treatment.

Microscopic evidence of endometriosis is always desirable but may be difficult to obtain. A biopsy diagnosis of endometriosis requires histological evidence of both endometrial glands and stroma. However, these characteristics are not always present in every biopsy, and biopsies may be difficult to obtain because implants overlie vital structures such as the bowel, bladder, or ureter. In a series of 74 patients with endoscopically proven endometriosis, Portuondo and coworkers [41] found that endometriosis could be confirmed by biopsy in only 72% of patients. The biopsy failures in this study were mainly related to technical difficulties of obtaining ovarian biopsies. Even at the time of laparotomy for conservative or definitive treatment for endometriosis, histological confirmation of endometriosis may be difficult. In cases where endometriosis may not be obvious to the pathologist, the surgeon should identify areas of endometriosis with a suture so that pathological sections can be taken of that specific area.

Second-look laparoscopy may be extremely useful in evaluating therapy for endometriosis. Laparoscopy performed within six months following surgery, as advocated by some, can evaluate the reformation of adhesions. Newly formed adhesions can often be lysed at this time before they become well organized and more vascular.

Constituents of Peritoneal Fluid

In studying the pathophysiology of endometriosis, the amount of peritoneal fluid and several of its constituents have been studied in search of information that would explain either the pathogenesis or the symptoms of this disease. Although patients with endometriosis have been reported to have an increase in the amount of peritoneal fluid, macrophages, and prostaglandins, these findings are inconsistent and not helpful in its diagnosis. Portuondo and coworkers [41] evaluated the usefulness of peritoneal flushing and aspiration in the early diagnosis of endometriosis. Of 74 patients with endometriosis, only 25% of the washings performed were successful in demonstrating endometrial glands or other evidence of endometriosis. There was no significant difference in peritoneal fluid characteristics or the exfoliative cytology in those patients with mild, moderate, or severe disease.

Since endometriosis may affect ovarian function, ovarian steroid hormones or other products in the peritoneal fluid could give information regarding whether or not ovarian dysfunction is present. Koninckx and associates [42] have studied peritoneal fluid steroid hormones and their binding proteins in patients with and without endometriosis. No difference was found in total protein, sex steroid hormone-binding protein, and transcortin concentrations. The concentrations of both progesterone and estradiol increased after ovulation in both groups of women, and the concentrations of estradiol and progesterone were not significantly different between these two groups of women except in women with unruptured but luteinized follicles. Patients with this syndrome, which seems to be more common in endometriosis patients, had lower concentrations of peritoneal fluid steroid hormones during the postovulatory period. Nevertheless, constituents of peritoneal fluid, including steroid hormones, are not helpful in the diagnosis of this disease.

Autoimmune Studies in Endometriosis

Recent work by several investigators support the hypothesis first proposed by Weed and Arquembourg [43] that "foreign" endometrial proteins present in the peritoneal cavity or at other sites could induce an autoimmune response that could be manifested either in the endometrium, peritoneal fluid, or the serum of patients with endometriosis. Alterations in the immune response have been suggested as a cause of infertility in women with endometriosis. Changes in the local level of immunoglobulins and sperm phagocytosis have been proposed as well as alterations in the systemic immune response. Endometriosis is thought to activate the complement system and to significantly alter complement components in serum, peritoneal fluid, and endometrium. It is also thought to increase the production of antibodies that may be found in increased concentrations in these same compartments.

For diagnostic purposes, studies may take the form of determining the presence of endometrial antibodies associated with the endometrium or in serum. Kreiner and coworkers [44] studied the presence of endometrial antibodies in endometrium by immunofluorescence in 18 patients with endometriosis documented at laparoscopy. Sixteen of these patients had positive immunofluorescence, indicating the presence of anti-IgG staining in the endometrium. However, of 24 patients with no evidence of endometriosis, 9 also exhibited immunofluorescence and 8 of these patients had evidence of pelvic inflammatory disease. If patients with either endometriosis or chronic pelvic inflammatory disease are studied, 96% will have positive tests for endometrial IgG. As a potential diagnostic test for either pelvic inflammatory disease or endometriosis, this test has a predictive value of 96%, 86% sensitivity, and 93% specificity for a positive test. A negative test was only 76% predictive of the absence of peritoneal disease. These data support the earlier work of Mathur et al. [45] and suggest that positive immunofluorescence of IgG binding in the endometrium may be a valuable predictor of laparoscopic findings and may be useful in the diagnosis of endometriosis or other pelvic diseases.

A screening test for antiendometrial antibodies in the serum of a patient with endometriosis would be even more valuable. Wild and Shivers [46] examined the sera of 42 patients complaining of infertility using an indirect immmunofluorescence for the presence of antibodies to the endometrium. The presence or absence of antibodies was matched with findings at the time of laparoscopy. Of 28 patients with positive antibody tests, 24 (85.7%) were found to have endometriosis. In this study, no correlation between the severity of endometriosis and the degree of immunofluorescence could be demonstrated. Further development of a noninvasive immunological test for the presence of endometriosis would not only be helpful in the diagnosis of this disorder but could be useful in monitoring the progress of disease with various treatment modalities.

A cell membrane antigen, CA-125, has been reported to be elevated in patients with endometriosis [47–49], but it also elevated in a variety of fetal and adult tissues as well as in several pathological disorders (see Chapter 3). It is not likely to be a specific marker for the diagnosis of endometriosis because it is also elevated in patients with inflammatory disease, ovarian carcinoma, and other pelvic disorders. However, it may be useful in monitoring the progress of disease following therapy.

Ultrasonography and Computerized Tomography

Ultrasonography and computerized tomography have been proposed to be helpful in the diagnosis and management of endometriosis. Certainly, these techniques are useful in confirming the presence of a pelvic mass, its size, and whether it changes significantly in size with time. But in the absence of a pelvic mass, the sensitivities of these techniques are in question. Several authors agree that endometriomas can be detected but cannot be differentiated from other cystic lesions of the ovaries or from pelvic inflammatory disease [50–54]. Friedman and associates [32] studied the effectiveness of ultrasound examination in the detection of endometriosis and found that ultrasound was successful in detecting endometriosis in only 4 of 37 patients (10.8%). These authors concluded that ultrasonography is neither sensitive nor specific in diagnosing endometriosis, and it does not have a role in the diagnosis or management of this disorder.

PITFALLS IN THE DIAGNOSIS OF ENDOMETRIOSIS

In the absence of a noninvasive diagnostic test for endometriosis, the diagnosis of this disorder must be based on its symptoms, physical findings, and direct visualization. As outlined by Dmowski [22], pitfalls do occur in the diagnosis of endometriosis, and many of these can be avoided. Although the prototype of the patient with endometriosis is the Caucasion woman who is underweight, overanxious, and career oriented, endometriosis can be found in any woman and should be highly suspected in patients with increasing dysmenorrhea and/or infertility. In any patient with infertility, even if the hysterosalpingogram is normal, endometriosis should be suspected and endoscopy performed. During laparoscopic evaluation, the pelvis should be systematically examined with attention to areas where endometriosis is commonly found. Laparoscopic findings frequently associated with endometriosis include peritoneal congestion, ovarian adhesions in the absence of obstructed fallopian tubes, peritoneal defects, ovaries adherent to the pelvic peritoneum, hemosiderin deposits, large amounts of serosanguineous peritoneal fluid, and atypical endometriotic lesions such as petechial hemorrhages or eccymotic implants associated with stellate scarring. Increased physician awareness of the subtle changes associated with endometriosis can enhance the chance of securing a diagnosis.

REFERENCES

1. Scott RB, Telinda RW: External endometriosis: The scourge of the private patient. Ann Surg 131:706, 1950.
2. Jenkins S, Olive DL, Haney AF: Endometriosis: pathogenic implications of the anatomic distribution. Obstet Gynecol 67:335, 1986.
3. Djursing H, Petersen K, Weberg E: Symptomatic postmenopausal endometriosis. Acta Obstet Scand 60:529, 1981.
4. Kempers RD, Dockerty MB, Hunt AB, Symmonds RE: Significant postmenopausal endometriosis surgery. Surg Gyn Obstet 11:348, 1960.
5. Shamshuddin AKM, Villa Santa U, Tang CK, Mohamed, NC: Adenocarcinoma arising from extragonadal endometriosis 14 years after total hysterectomy and bilateral salpingo-oophorectomy for endometriosis. Am J Obstet Gynecol 133:585, 1979.
6. Hertig AT, Gore H: Tumors of the female sex organs (pt 3). Tumors of the ovary and fallopian tubes. In "Atlas of Tumor Pathology." Armed Forces Institute of Pathology, 1961.
7. Cohen MR: Laparoscopy: diagnostic and surgical. In Givens JR (ed): "The Infertile Female." Chicago: Year Book Medical Publishers, p 483, 1979.
8. Moon YS, Leung PCS, Yuen BH, Gomel V: Prostaglandin F in human endometriosis tissue. Am J Obstet Gynecol 141:344, 1981.
9. Ferrlira SH, Mondaco S, Vane JR: Prostaglandins and signs and symptoms of inflammation . In Robinson HJ, Vane JR (eds): "Protaglandin Synthetase Inhibitors." New York: Raven Press, p 175, 1974.
10. Singh EJ, Baccarini IM, Zuspan FP: Levels of prostaglandins F2 and E2 in human endometrium during the menstrual cycle. Am J Obstet Gynecol 121:1003, 1975.
11. Kauipilla A, Poulakka J, Ylikorkala O: Prostaglandin biosynthesis inhibitors and endometriosis. Prostaglandins 18:655, 1979.

12. Porina M, Vespasiani G, Vergill G, Mearini E, Micali F: Ureteral endometriosis: an endoscopic diagnosis. Urology 26:566, 1985.
13. Klein RS, Cattolica EV: Ureteral endometriosis. Urology 13:477, 1979.
14. Kerr WS: Endometriosis involving the urinary tract. Clin Obstet Gynecol 9:331, 1966.
15. Rosenberg SK, Jacobs H: Endometriosis of the upper ureter. Urology 121:512, 1979.
16. Egger H, Weigmann P: Clinical and surgical aspects of ovarian endometriotic cysts. Arch Gynecol 233:37, 1982.
17. Husson HM: Incidence of endometriosis in diagnostic laparascopy. J Reprod Med 16:135, 1976.
18. Medega C, Marchesini FP, Bellettini L, Biscontin S, Flamigni C: Diagnostic value of laparoscopy in endometriosis and infertility. J Reprod Med 29:597, 1984.
19. Cramer DW, Wilson E, Stillman RJ, Berger MJ, Belisle S, Schiff I, Albrecht B, Gibson M, Stodel B, Schoenbaum SC: The relation of endometriosis to menstrual characteristics, smoking and exercise. JAMA 255:1904, 1986.
20. Wilson EA, Osbourne L, Vernon MW: Menstrual characteristics of patients with endometriosis. Infertility 9:71, 1986.
21. Wentz AC: Premenstrual spotting: its association with endometriosis but not luteal phase inadequacy. Fertil Steril 33:605, 1980.
22. Dmowski WP: Pitfalls in clinical, laparoscopic and histologic diagnosis of endometriosis. Acta Obstet Gynecol Scand (Suppl) 123:61, 1984.
23. Muse KN, Wilson EA: How does mild endometriosis cause infertility? Fertil Steril 38:145, 1982.
24. Petersohn L: Fertility in patients with ovarian endometriosis before and after treatment. Acta Obstet Gynecol Scand 49:331, 1970.
25. Rock JA, Guzick DS, Sengos C, Schweditsch M, Sapp KC, Jones HW Jr.: The conservative treatment of endometriosis: evaluation of pregnancy success with respect to the extent of disease as categorized using contemporary classification systems. Fertil Steril 35:131, 1981.
26. Naples JD, Batt RE, Sadigh H: Spontaneous abortion rate in patients with endometriosis. Obstet Gynecol 57:509, 1981.
27. Wheeler JM, Johnston BM, Malinak LR: The relationship of endometriosis to spontaneous abortion: effect of control group selection. Fertil Steril 39:656, 1983.
28. Metzger DA, Olive DL, Stohs GF, Franklin RR: Association of endometriosis and spontaneous abortion: effect of control group selection. Fertil Steril 46:18, 1986.
29. Frey GH: The familial occurrence of endometriosis. Am J Obstet Gynecol 73:418, 1957.
30. Ranney B: Endometriosis: IV: hereditary tendency. Obstet Gynecol 37:734, 1970.
31. Simpson JL, Elias S, Malinak LR, Bertram VC: Heritable aspects of endometriosis: I: genetic studies. Am J Obstet Gynecol 137:327, 1980.
32. Friedman H, Vogelzang RL, Mendelson EB, Neiman HL, Cohen M: Endometriosis detection by US with laparoscopic correlation. Radiology 157:217, 1985.
33. Majmudar B, Henderson PH III, Semple E: Salpingitis isthmica nodosa: a high-risk factor for tubal pregnancy. Obstet Gynecol 62:73, 1983.
34. Karasick S, Karasick D, Shilling J: Salpingitis isthmica nodosa in female infertility. J Assoc Canad Radiol 36:188, 1985.
35. Mills J, Upadhayay PP, Carstairs LS: Diverticulosis of the fallopian tubes - salpingitis isthmica nodosa. Clinic Radiol 19:233, 1968.
36. Elmahgoub S: Progestin treatment of uterotubal (Cornual) block. Int J Gynecol Obstet 16:303, 1979.

37. Salat-Baroux T, Cornier E, Coutrier JY: Obstruction pathologique de la partion initiale di isthme tubaire analyse de 50 interventions microchirurgicales. J Gynecol Obstet Biol Reprod 9:63, 1980.
38. Drake TS, Grunert GM: The unsuspected pelvic factor in the infertility investigation. Fertil Steril 34:27, 1980.
39. Vernon MW, Beard JS, Graves K, Wilson E: Classification of endrometriotic implants by morphologic appearance and capacity to synthesize prostaglandin F. Fertil Steril. In Press.
40. Chatman, DL: Pelvic peritoneal defects and endometriosis: Allan-Masters syndrome revisited. Fertil Steril 34:27, 1980.
41. Portuondo JA, Herran C, Echanojaurequi AD, Riego AG: Peritoneal flushing and biopsy in laparoscopically diagnosed endometriosis. Fertil Steril 38:538, 1982.
42. Koninckx PR, Ide P, Vandenbroucke W, Brosens IA: New aspects of the pathophysiology of endometriosis and associated infertility. J Reprod Med 24:257, 1980.
43. Weed JC, Arquembourg PC: Endometriosis: can it produce an antoimmmune response resulting in infertility? Clin Obstet Gynecol 23:885, 1980.
44. Kreiner D, Fromowitz FB, Richardson DA, Kenigsberg D: Endometrial immunofluorescence associated with endometriosis and pelvic inflammatory disease. Fertil Steril 46:243, 1986.
45. Mathur S, Peress MR, Williamson HO, Youmans CD, Maney SA, Garvin AJ, Rust PF, Fundenberg HH: Autoimmunity to endometrium and ovary in endometriosis. Clin Exp Immunol 50:259, 1982.
46. Wild RA, Shivers CA: Antiendometrial antibodies in patients with endometriosis. Am J Reprod Immunol Microbiol 8:84, 1985.
47. Niloff JM, Knapp RC, Schnaetzl E, Reynolds C, Bast RC Jr: CA-125 antigen levels in obstetric and gynecological patients. Obstet Gynecol 64:703, 1984.
48. Barbieri RL, Niloff JM, Bast RC Jr., Schnaetzl E, Kistner RW, Knapp RC: Elevated serum concentrations of CA-125 in patients with advanced endometriosis. Fertil Steril 45:630, 1986.
49. Guidice LC, Jacobs A, Pineda J, Bell CE, Lippman L: Serum levels of CA-125 in patients with endometriosis. Fertil Steril 45:876, 1986.
50. Coleman BG, Arger PH, Mulbern CG: Endometriosis: clinical and ultrasonic correlation. AJR 132:747, 1979.
51. Walsh JW, Taylor KJW, Rosenfield AT: Gray scale ultrasonography in the diagnosis of endometriosis and adenomyosis. AJR 132:87, 1979.
52. Haulsins AJ, Goodwin WP, Ervin CW, Mitchell DP: Pelvic endometriosis as demonstrated by gray scale ultrasound. J Nat Med Assn 71:289, 1979.
53. Sandler MA, Karo JJ: The spectrum of ultrasonic findings in endometriosis. Radiology 127:299, 1978.
54. Fishman EK, Scatarige JC, Saksouk FA, Rosenshein NB, Siegelman SS: Computed tomography of endometriosis. J Comput Assist Tomogr 76:257, 1983.

Endometriosis, pages 79–89

Chapter 5
Classification of Endometriosis

Emery A. Wilson, M.D.

Division of Reproductive Endocrinology and Infertility, Kentucky Center for Reproductive Medicine, University of Kentucky College of Medicine, Lexington, Kentucky 40536

INTRODUCTION

Prior to development of classification schemes for endometriosis, pregnancy rates following therapy for endometriosis varied widely. In a review [1] of the pregnancy rates following conservative surgery for endometriosis prior to 1971, the results varied from 13% to 94%. Much of the disparity in pregnancy rates reported by these authors was based on the differences in severity of disease and, without a classification system, the wide range in pregnancy rates was difficult to interpret.

EVOLUTION OF ENDOMETRIOSIS CLASSIFICATIONS

The first attempt to classify endometriosis was in 1961 by Riva, Wilson, and Kawasaki [2], who proposed a simple method of classifying endometriosis in order to objectively study the effects of norethynodrel as a form of medical therapy. This classification was arbitrarily based on the number of pelvic structures involved, with paired organs such as the tubes or ovaries considered separately. The disease was listed as minimal if one to three structures were involved, moderate if four to six structures were involved, and severe if seven or more organs were affected. This classification system was used to evaluate the effects of medical therapy only in this study but was never really proposed for use by other physicians.

The first classification system to be offered for universal use was proposed by Beecham in 1966 [3] to keep accurate records on the progress of endometriosis and to record the response to endocrine therapy. The classification had four stages varying from scattered small endometriosis implants to massive involvement, but stages two through four could be used to describe either the palpable findings on physical examination or the findings at operation. Thus, the severity of disease and the associated classification was not based on direct visualization or biopsy-proven endometriosis.

Credit for the establishment and continued emphasis of a classification of endometriosis goes to the group at Baylor College of Medicine, who have long had an interest in standardizing the severity and treatment of this disorder. In order to establish and document the premise that the degree of infertility in women with endometriosis was dependent on the severity of the disease, a classification of endometriosis was established known as the Acosta Classification (Table I). Acosta and coworkers [4] proposed a classification of pelvic endometriosis based on a study of 107 infertile patients who underwent conservative operative treatment of endometriosis. The classification was separated into three categories: mild, moderate, and severe. Mild endometriosis consisted of scattered endometriosis implants but no periovarian or peritubal adhesions. Moderate endometriosis consisted of small endometriomas (less than 2 cm) or the presence of minimal periovarian or

TABLE I. Acosta Classification of Pelvic Endometriosis

Classification	Characteristics
Mild	1) Scattered, fresh lesions (i.e., implants not associated with scarring or retraction of the peritoneum) in the anterior or posterior cul-de-sac or pelvic peritoneum. 2) Rare surface implant on ovary, with no endometrioma, without surface scarring and retraction and without periovarian adhesions. 3) No peritubular adhesions.
Moderate	1) Endometriosis involving one or both ovaries, with several surface lesions, with scarring and retraction or small endometriomata. 2) Minimal periovarian adhesions associated with ovarian lesions described. 3) Minimal peritubular adhesions associated with ovarian lesions described. 4) Superficial implants in the anterior and/or posterior cul-de-sac with scarring and retraction. Some adhesions, but not sigmoid invasion.
Severe	1) Endometriosis involving one or both ovaries with endometrioma $> 2 \times 2$ cm (usually both). 2) One or both ovaries bound down by adhesions associated with endometriosis, with or without tubal adhesions to ovaries. 3) One or both tubes bound down or obstructed by endometriosis; associated adhesions or lesions. 4) Obliteration of the cul-de-sac from adhesions or lesions associated with endometriosis. 5) Thickening of the uterosacral ligaments and cul-de-sac lesions from invasive endometriosis with obliteration of the cul-de-sac. 6) Significant bowel or urinary tract involvement.

peritubal adhesions. Severe disease included those patients with large endometriomas, extensive adhesive disease, tubal obstruction, and obliteration of the cul-de-sac by adhesions associated with endometriosis. The appropriateness of the Acosta classification was confirmed by the postoperative pregnancy rates of 75% for mild disease, 50% for moderate disease, and 33% for severe disease. This was the first classification system to be universally accepted, because it not only depicted the severity of disease but it also could be used to provide a prognosis for fertility.

The advantage of the Acosta system was that it was relatively uncomplicated and easy to remember. Although the Acosta classification was helpful for both documenting the severity of disease and pregnancy prognosis, the differences between stages were nonspecific and many patients did not fall into the assigned categories [1]. For example, the Acosta classification did not distinguish between unilateral and bilateral disease. Presumably, pregnancy would be more likely when only one adnexa was involved. Furthermore, to assign a patient to moderate disease or severe disease based on the presence of an ovarian endometrioma of 2 cm or more was thought to be arbitrary.

In 1977, Kistner, Siegler, and Behrman suggested another classification for endometriosis that was based, to a certain degree, on the natural history of the disease [5]. This classification system was much more extensive but also nonspecific in that the presence of unilateral or bilateral disease was not taken into consideration.

Because none of these classifications attained general acceptance by clinicians, the American Fertility Society published its first classification system in 1979 [6]. This classification was based on a point system to determine the stage or degree of severity of endometriosis. The basis of the classification was the natural progression of the disease with allowances made for unilateral involvement. According to this classification, endometriosis was divided into four stages based on the accumulation of points arbitrarily assigned to the presence and extent of endometriosis implants, adhesions, endometriomas, and tubal occlusion: mild (1 to 5 points), moderate (6 to 15 points), severe (16 to 30 points), and extensive (31 to 54 points).

The American Fertility Society classification of endometriosis and its acceptance by most clinicians clearly improved the classification for this disease. The medical and surgical treatment of the disease could be evaluated and various forms of therapy could be compared between institutions. However, the value of this classification system has probably been studied more objectively than previous systems, and it was also found to be inadequate.

Hasson [7] emphasized that the classification system did not take into consideration the three-dimensional volumetric assessment of the endometriotic lesions. Rock and coworkers [8] and Guzick and associates [9] retrospectively studied the efficacy of the American Fertility Society classification of endometriosis and found that it effectively categorized the severity of disease but that each classification category was arbitrarily assigned point scores that may not reflect true relative risk and that the point scores that separated the various stages were arbitrarily chosen. In addition, the classification was not very helpful in predicting whether patients would need subsequent surgery except when there was extensive disease. Kable and Yussman [10] found that the stage of disease had no prognostic effect on the pregnancy rate following therapy. Although the results of these studies differ from previous reports, they emphasize the arbitrary point assignment and categories in the American Fertility Society classification. Finally, Brosens et al. [11] reported that the classification had been a useful tool for evaluating the efficacy of surgical management of endometriosis, but could be misused in evaluating the efficacy of medical treatment and was inadequate for staging the milder degrees of endometriosis. These authors emphasized that the size and extent of peritoneal implants may be important and this could be best evaluated by biopsy. These authors also emphasized that the hormonal status of the patient at the time of observation was important.

Thus, the need for revisions in the American Fertility Society classification of endometriosis became necessary.

REVISED AMERICAN FERTILITY SOCIETY CLASSIFICATION OF ENDOMETRIOSIS

Because of the criticism outlined above with the first American Fertility Society classification, a revised classification was reported in 1985 [12]. The revised classification is presented in Figure 1 and examples of each stage are presented in Figure 2.

The revised classification also uses a point system for staging endometriosis. It differs from the previous classification by adding a category for minimal disease and eliminating the category for extensive disease. Greater attention is given to the differences between peritoneal and ovarian endometriosis as well as to the depth of invasion of endometriosis into the peritoneum and ovaries. Complete obliteration of the cul-de-sac is considered a poor prognostic sign for fertility, and the presence of this finding automatically places the patient in the severe category.

The Revised American Fertility Society Classification of Endometriosis is not without criticism. For example, if the classification is to provide a prognosis for fertility, the number of points assigned to tubal occlusion or

THE AMERICAN FERTILITY SOCIETY
REVISED CLASSIFICATION OF ENDOMETRIOSIS

Patient's Name ______________________________ Date ______________________

Stage I (Minimal) - 1-5
Stage II (Mild) - 6-15
Stage III (Moderate) - 16-40
Stage IV (Severe) - >40
Total ____________

Laparoscopy ________ Laparotomy ________ Photography ________
Recommended Treatment ______________________________
____
Prognosis ______________

PERITONEUM	ENDOMETRIOSIS	< 1cm	1-3cm	> 3cm
	Superficial	1	2	4
	Deep	2	4	6
OVARY	R Superficial	1	2	4
	Deep	4	16	20
	L Superficial	1	2	4
	Deep	4	16	20
	POSTERIOR CULDESAC OBLITERATION	Partial		Complete
		4		40
OVARY	ADHESIONS	< 1/3 Enclosure	1/3-2/3 Enclosure	> 2/3 Enclosure
	R Filmy	1	2	4
	Dense	4	8	16
	L Filmy	1	2	4
	Dense	4	8	16
TUBE	R Filmy	1	2	4
	Dense	4*	8*	16
	L Filmy	1	2	4
	Dense	4*	8*	16

*If the fimbriated end of the fallopian tube is completely enclosed, change the point assignment to 16.

Additional Endometriosis: ______________________________

Associated Pathology: ______________________________

To Be Used with Normal Tubes and Ovaries

L R

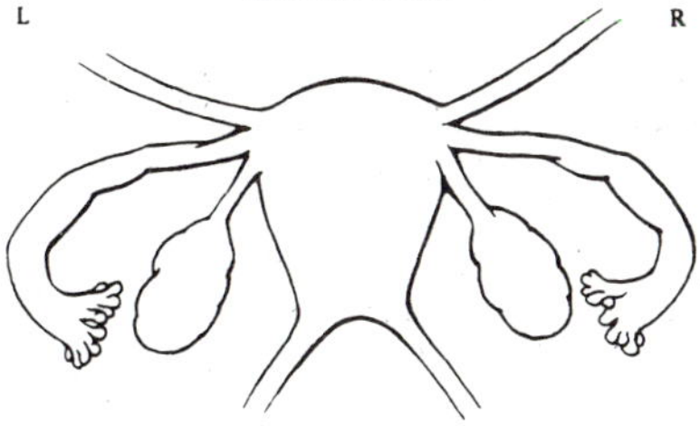

To Be Used with Abnormal Tubes and/or Ovaries

L R

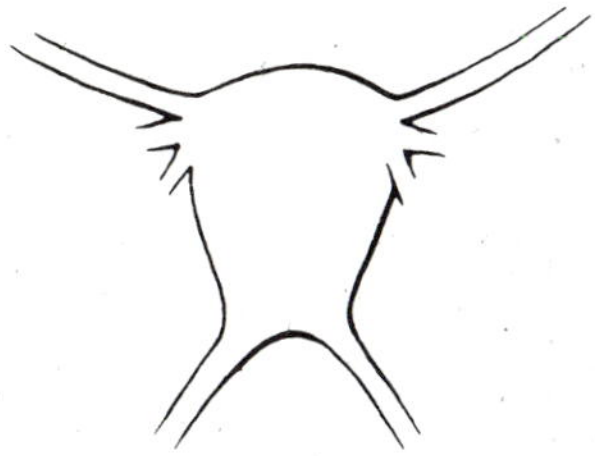

Fig. 1. Revised American Fertility Society Classification for Endometriosis. Reproduced with the permission of the publisher, The American Fertility Society.

EXAMPLES & GUIDELINES

STAGE I (MINIMAL)

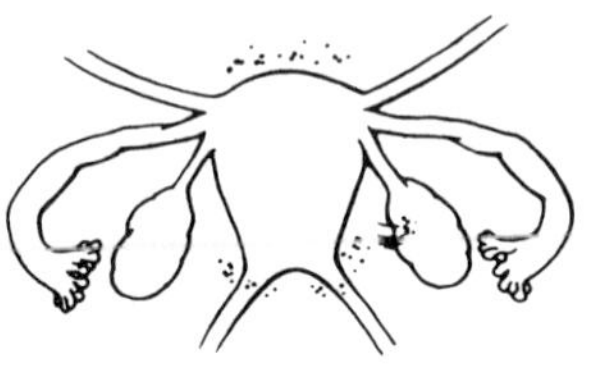

PERITONEUM			
Superficial Endo	–	1-3cm	- 2
R. OVARY			
Superficial Endo	–	< 1cm	- 1
Filmy Adhesions	–	< 1/3	- 1
TOTAL POINTS			4

STAGE II (MILD)

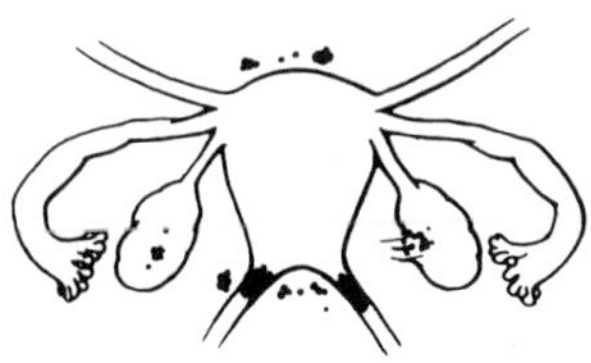

PERITONEUM			
Deep Endo	–	> 3cm	- 6
R. OVARY			
Superficial Endo	–	< 1cm	- 1
Filmy Adhesions	–	< 1/3	- 1
L. OVARY			
Superficial Endo	–	< 1cm	- 1
TOTAL POINTS			9

STAGE III (MODERATE)

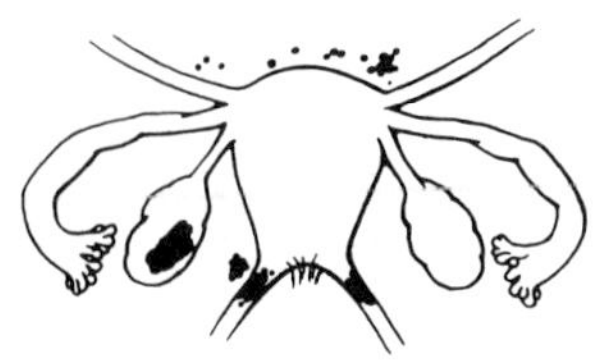

PERITONEUM			
Deep Endo	–	> 3cm	- 6
CULDESAC			
Partial Obliteration			- 4
L. OVARY			
Deep Endo	–	1-3cm	- 16
TOTAL POINTS			26

STAGE III (MODERATE)

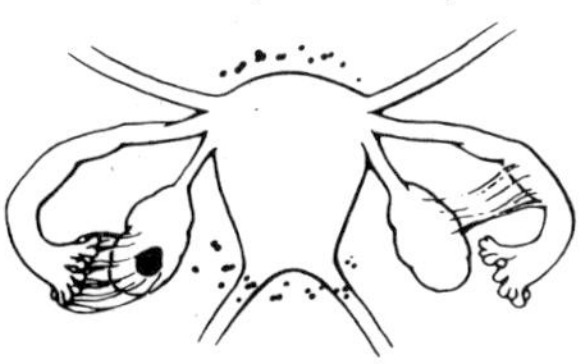

PERITONEUM			
Superficial Endo	–	> 3cm	- 3
R. TUBE			
Filmy Adhesions	–	< 1/3	- 1
R. OVARY			
Filmy Adhesions	–	< 1/3	- 1
L. TUBE			
Dense Adhesions	–	< 1/3	- 16*
L. OVARY			
Deep Endo	–	< 1 cm	-4
Dense Adhesions	–	< 1/3	-4
TOTAL POINTS			29

STAGE IV (SEVERE)

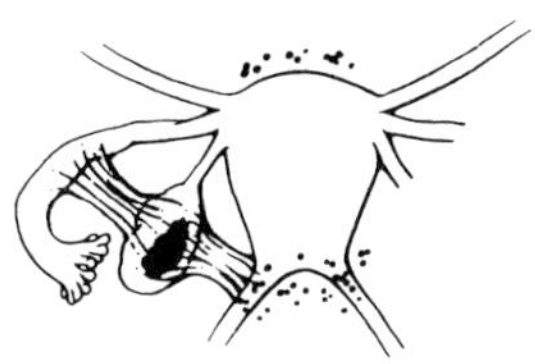

PERITONEUM			
Superficial Endo	–	> 3cm	- 3
L. OVARY			
Deep Endo	–	1-3cm	- 32**
Dense Adhesions	–	< 1/3	- 8**
L. TUBE			
Dense Adhesions	–	< 1/3	-8**
TOTAL POINTS			51

*Point assignment changed to 16

**Point assignment doubled

STAGE IV (SEVERE)

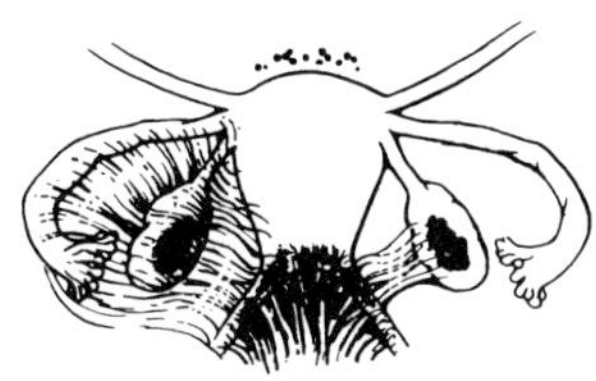

PERITONEUM			
Deep Endo	–	> 3cm	- 6
CULDESAC			
Complete Obliteration			- 40
R. OVARY			
Deep Endo	–	1-3cm	- 16
Dense Adhesions	–	< 1/3	- 4
L. TUBE			
Dense Adhesions	–	> 2/3	- 16
L. OVARY			
Deep Endo	–	1-3cm	- 16
Dense Adhesions	–	> 2/3	- 16
TOTAL POINTS			114

Determination of the stage or degree of endometrial involvement is based on a weighted point system. Distribution of points has been arbitrarily determined and may require further revision or refinement as knowledge of the disease increases.

To ensure complete evaluation, inspection of the pelvis in a clockwise or counterclockwise fashion is encouraged. Number, size and location of endometrial implants, plaques, endometriomas and/or adhesions are noted. For example, five separate 0.5cm superficial implants on the peritoneum (2.5 cm total) would be assigned 2 points. (The surface of the uterus should be considered peritoneum.) The severity of the endometriosis or adhesions should be assigned the highest score only for peritoneum, ovary, tube or culdesac. For example, a 4cm superficial and a 2cm deep implant of the peritoneum should be given a score of 6 (not 7). A 4cm deep endometrioma of the ovary associated with more than 3cm of superficial disease should be scored 20 (not 24).

In those patients with only one adenexa, points applied to disease of the remaining tube and ovary should be multipled by two. **Points assigned may be circled and totaled. Aggregation of points indicates stage of disease (minimal, mild, moderate, or severe).

The presence of endometriosis of the bowel, urinary tract, fallopian tube, vagina, cervix, skin etc., should be documented under "additional endometriosis." Other pathology such as tubal occlusion, leiomyomata, uterine anomaly, etc., should be documented under "associated pathology." All pathology should be depicted as specifically as possible on the sketch of pelvic organs, and means of observation (laparoscopy or laparotomy) should be noted.

Fig. 2. Examples of various stages of endometriosis according to the Revised American Fertility Society classification. Reproduced with the permission of the publisher, The American Fertility Society.

3

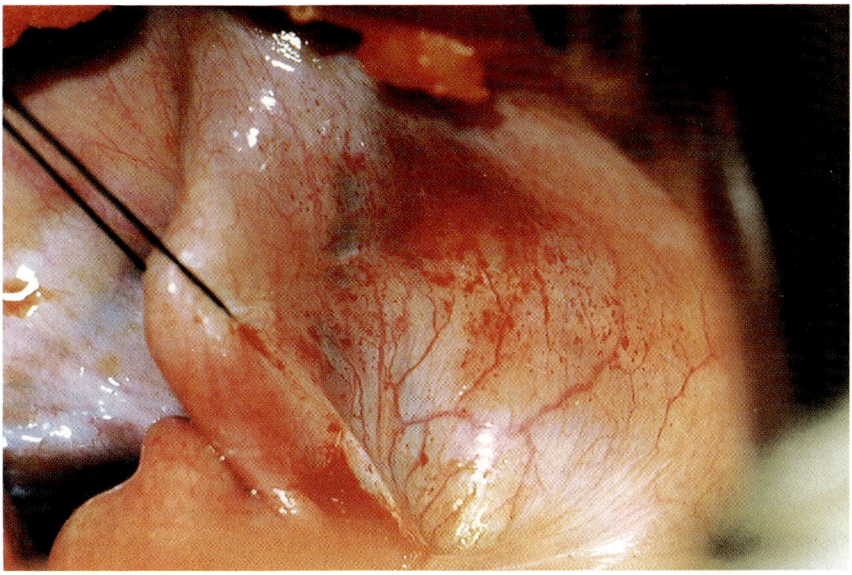

4

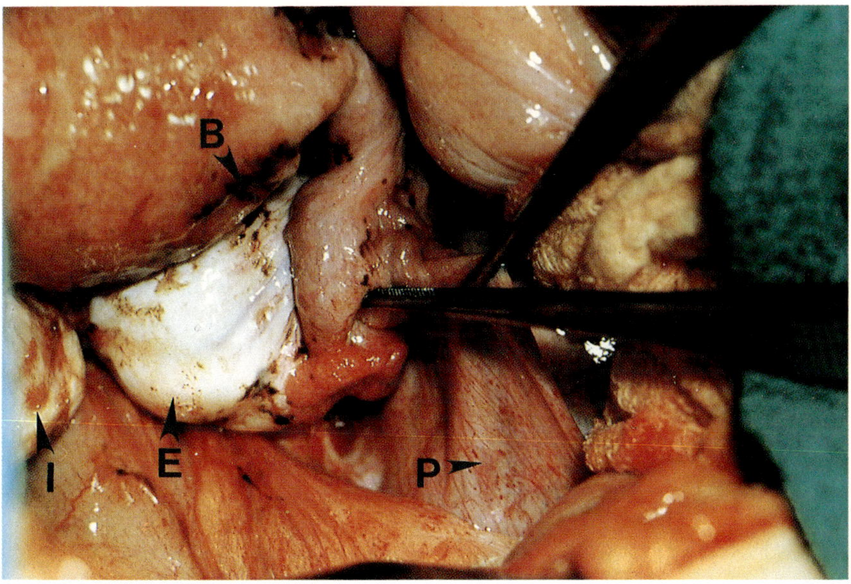

Fig. 3. Petechial implants characteristic of early endometriosis anterior to the round ligament (suture).

Fig. 4. Severe endometriosis in a patient undergoing definitive surgery: petechial implants (P), intermediate implants (I), powder-burn implants (B), and endometrioma (E). Note the fimbria of the oviduct, which is usually patent.

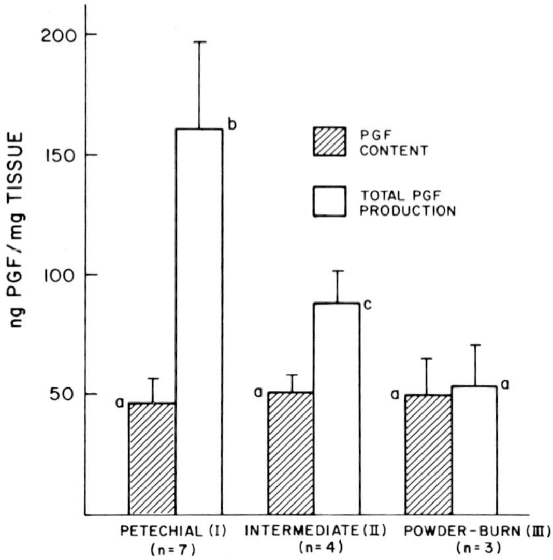
200
150
100
50
ng PGF / mg TISSUE
PGF
CONTENT
TOTAL PGF
PRODUCTION
a
b
a
c
a
a
PETECHIAL (I)
(n=7)
INTERMEDIATE (II)
(n=4)
POWDER-BURN (III)
(n=3)

5

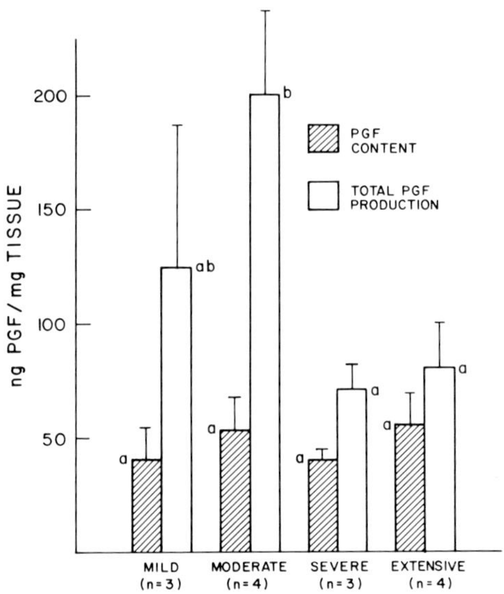
200
150
100
50
ng PGF / mg TISSUE
PGF
CONTENT
TOTAL PGF
PRODUCTION
a
ab
a
b
a
a
a
a
MILD
(n=3)
MODERATE
(n=4)
SEVERE
(n=3)
EXTENSIVE
(n=4)

6

enclosure of the fimbriated end of the fallopian tube with adhesions may be inadequate. Theoretically, if both fallopian tubes were completely enclosed and no other signs of endometriosis were present, a patient would have absolute infertility and yet be assigned 32 points, which would place her only in the moderate category of disease. Continued revisions of the classification system may be necessary and are anticipated as more knowledge is obtained regarding endometriosis and as this classification system is evaluated [1]. Brosens and coworkers [11] have emphasized the need for physiopathologic as well as the descriptive considerations for the classifications of uncomplicated endometriosis. In other words, the biochemical or functional nature of the endometriotic implant may be more significant than the extent of disease or the degree of adhesion formation.

PATHOPHYSIOLOGIC CATEGORIES OF ENDOMETRIOSIS

The inconsistencies between the severity of symptoms and the extent of disease as depicted by previous classification systems suggest that additional subtle interactions may be present in patients with endometriosis that cannot be fully explained by the physical attributes used in current classification systems. Lack of correlation between symptoms and severity of disease may be due to variations in the metabolic activity of endometriosis implants present at different stages of disease. The classification of endometriosis has been based primarily on size and location of implants as well as the magnitude of adhesion formation and involvement of other organ systems. However, the biochemical viability or the morphologic appearance of endometriosis

---

Fig. 5. Content and in vitro production of prostaglandin F by endometriosis implants classified by gross and histologic appearance. Each bar represents the mean $\pm$ SEM and the bars with common alphabetical letters are not statistically different ($p < 0.05$). From Vernon MW, Beard JS, Graves KL, Wilson EA: Classification of endometriotic implants by morphologic appearance and capacity to synthesize prostaglandin F. Fertil Steril 46:801, 1986. Reproduced with the permission of the publisher, The American Fertility Society, Birmingham, AL.

Fig. 6. Content and in vitro production of prostaglandin F by endometriosis implants from patients classified according to severity of endometriosis. The stages are defined according to the 1979 American Fertility Society classification. Each bar represents the mean $\pm$ SEM and the bars with common alphabetical letters are not statistically different ($p < 0.05$). From Vernon MW, Beard JS, Graves KL, Wilson EA: Classification of endometriotic implants by morphologic appearance and capacity to synthesize protaglandin F. Fertil Steril 46:801, 1986. Reproduced with the permission of the publisher, The American Fertility Society, Birmingham, AL.

implants have not yet been incorporated into schemes for classifying endometriosis. The variability between the severity of symptoms and the extent of disease may be a result of the functional status of the implant.

The endometrium is known to be metabolically alive in the production of substances that could modify the symptoms associated with endometriosis. The endometrium is known, for example, to produce large concentrations of prostaglandins, particularly prostaglandin F, and prostaglandins are also known to be produced by endometriosis implants [13,14].

Vernon and coworkers [14] have proposed a classification of endometriosis based on the morphological appearance of endometriosis implants and their capacity to synthesize prostaglandins. Endometriosis implants were categorized into three morphological appearances: red, petechial implants; reddish-brown, intermediate implants; and dark brown, "powder burn" implants (See Figs. 3 and 4). Although the prostaglandin content was similar for all three types of implants, petechial implants synthesized significantly more prostaglandin F than intermediate implants, which in turn synthesized more prostaglandins than the "powder burn" implants (Fig. 5). Although the "powder burn" implants contained prostaglandin F, this tissue did not have the capacity for de novo synthesis of prostaglandins. This information implies that the appearance of implants and their capacity to secrete products such as prostaglandins, which could cause symptoms or interfere with fertility, may be as important as the criteria that are currently used in classification systems.

The importance of the functional capacity of endometriosis was further emphasized when prostaglandin secretion by endometriotic implants were classified according to stage of disease (Fig. 6). The implants of patients with severe or extensive endometriosis did not produce more prostaglandins than they contained, whereas implants from patients with mild and moderate endometriosis produced five times more prostaglandins than they contained. Since prostaglandins are known to mediate tubal and uterine motility, ovulation, and possibly luteolysis, it is quite possible that the metabolic products of endometriosis implants could be responsible for reproductive dysfunction as well as other symptoms associated with this disease.

Further revisions of the American Fertility Society classification of endometriosis may well include studies on the morphological appearance of endometrial implants as well as their metabolic activity.

REFERENCES

1. Buttram VC: Evolution of the Revised American Fertility Society Classification of Endometriosis. Fertil Steril 43:347, 1985.

2. Riva HS, Wilson JH, Kawasaki DM: Effect of norethynodrel on endometriosis. Am J Obstet Gynecol 82:109, 1961.
3. Beecham CT: Classification of endometriosis. Obstet Gynecol 28:437, 1966.
4. Acosta AA, Buttram VC, Besch PK, Malinak R, Franklin RR, Vanderheyden JD: A proposed classification of pelvic endometriosis. Obstet Gynecol 42:19, 1973.
5. Kistner RW, Siegler AM, Behrman SJ: Suggested classification for endometriosis: relationship to infertility. Fertil Steril 28:1008, 1977.
6. The American Fertility Society: classification of endometriosis. Fertil Steril 32:633, 1979.
7. Hasson HM: Classification for endometriosis. Fertil Steril 35:368, 1981.
8. Rock JA, Guzick DS, Sengos C, Schweditsch M, Sapp KC, Jones HJ: The conservative surgical treatment of endometriosis: evaluation of pregnancy success with respect to the extent of disease as categorized using contemporary classification systems. Fertil Steril 35:131, 1981.
9. Guzick DS, Bross DS, Rock JA: Assessing the efficacy of The American Fertility Society's classification of endometriosis: application of a dose-response methodology. Fertil Steril 38:171, 1982.
10. Kable WT, Yussman MA: Fertility after conservative treatment of endometriosis. J Reprod Med 30:857, 1985.
11. Brosens IA, Cornillie F, Koninckx P, Vasquez G: Evolution of the revised American Fertility Society classification of endometriosis. Fertil Steril 44:714, 1985.
12. The American Fertility Society: Revised American Fertility Society classification of endometriosis: 1985. Fertil Steril 43:351, 1985.
13. Moon YS, Leung PCS, Yuen BH, Gomel V: Prostaglandin F in human endometriosis tissue. Am J Obstet Gynecol 141:344, 1981.
14. Vernon MW, Beard J, Graves KL, Wilson EA: Classification of endometriotic implants by morphological appearance and capacity to synthesize prostaglandin F. Fertil Steril 46:801, 1986.

Endometriosis, pages 91–110

Chapter 6
Endometriosis and Infertility

Ken Muse, M.D.

Kentucky Center for Reproductive Medicine, Division of Reproductive Endocrinology, Department of Obstetrics and Gynecology, University of Kentucky Medical Center, Lexington, Kentucky 40536-0084

INTRODUCTION

The hallmark of endometriosis is infertility. Exact epidemiologic data describing endometriosis and endometriosis-associated infertility do not exist, but it is generally agreed that 30% to 40% of patients with endometriosis are infertile (twice the rate of infertility in the general population [1]) and that 6% to 15% of infertile patients have endometriosis as their only identifiable infertility factor [2]. Despite its obvious importance, the mechanism by which endometriosis causes decreased fertility is not known.

Although a direct cause-and-effect relationship between endometriosis and infertility is not seriously doubted, the clinical manifestations of this link are quite variable. Many women with endometriosis have normal fertility, and, conversely, women with very minimal endometriosis may have severe and intractable symptoms, including infertility. In general, however, the decrement in fertility correlates roughly with the amount of disease present (number and size of the endometriosis lesions, and extent of adhesions and tissue destruction due to the disease) [3]. A variety of "staging" systems have been developed to quantitate endometriosis in a given patient [4], but their prognostic value is poorly defined [5].

INFERTILITY IN SEVERE DISEASE

The cause of infertility in women with severe endometriosis is easy to understand, intuitively. By definition, these women have extensive pelvic adhesions, distortion of tubo-ovarian relationships, and even destruction of some ovarian or tubal tissues. Ovulation, ovum pickup, and fertilization are mechanically hindered. Although commonly assumed to result from menstruation within the implants and secondary inflammation, little experimental evidence supports this idea, and the mechanism by which endometriosis causes adhesions and tissue damage is unknown. The reason for wide differences in observed adhesion formation between patients with similar degrees of endometriosis is also a mystery.

INFERTILITY IN MILD DISEASE

In women who have minimal endometriosis as their only discernible cause for infertility, the mechanism of their lessened fertility is obscure. Certain clinical data suggest that such a cause and effect may not exist. Olive and Haney [6], in a review of available treatments for endometriosis-associated infertility, concluded that no treatment had been shown to be superior to expectant management in patients with minimal disease. Schenken and Malinak [7] found surgical treatment to be of little benefit in this instance, as did Butler et al. [8] and Seibel et al. [9] with regard to medical (danazol) therapy. Regardless of treatment, most women eventually became pregnant, suggesting that the disease may play a coincidental or trivial role in fertility.

Convincing data that minimal endometriosis interferes with fertility come from other studies. In examining the success rate of donor insemination, Jansen [10] found that the presence of mild endometriosis decreased the chances for pregnancy in otherwise normal women; Hammond et al. [11] confirmed these results and found that danazol treatment improved pregnancy rates in these patients. In laparoscopic studies of endometriosis in fertile and infertile women, Strathy and coworkers were also able to link endometriosis and infertility [12].

This chapter examines the various theories that have arisen to explain endometriosis-associated infertility, and the evidence for and against each one (Table I). The extensive literature arising from animal models of endometriosis is mentioned only when particularly important, as this information is discussed in Chapter 12.

ABNORMAL PERITONEAL FLUID

In normal women with regular menstrual cycles, approximately 5 ml of peritoneal fluid is present in the pelvis during the follicular phase of the cycle. Immediately before and after ovulation, this fluid increases to approximately 20 ml, a combined result of ovarian transudate and steroid-rich follicular fluid. Various components in the fluid from endometriosis patients have been investigated for antifertility properties (Fig. 1).

TABLE I. Proposed Mechanisms for Endometriosis-Associated Infertility

Peritoneal fluid
Direct toxic effects
Prostaglandins
Macrophages
Immune dysfunction
Ovarian dysfunction
Anovulation
Luteal phase inadequacy
LUFS
Abnormal LH surge
Prolactin excess
Spontaneous abortions
Hereditary factors

Direct Toxic Effects

Morcos et al. [13] and Gerrity and coworkers [14] found that peritoneal fluid from infertile women with endometriosis was toxic to the growth and development of mouse embryos, when compared to the fluid from normal women and infertile women without endometriosis. Similarly, Sueldo and colleagues [15] found that peritoneal fluid from infertile endometriosis patients was more detrimental to the mouse sperm-ova interaction than was peritoneal fluid from control women. Using the human sperm penetration of zona-free hamster ova test, Halme and Hall [16] saw no difference in results between heat-treated peritoneal fluid from normal and endometriosis women. Chacho and coworkers [17] found that media used to incubate peritoneal macrophages did interfere with sperm-egg interaction in this system, however. Muse et al. [18] examined sperm motility in peritoneal fluid from women with and without endometriosis, and found no difference between the two groups.

Taken together, these studies suggest that unidentified factors may be present in the peritoneal fluid of endometriosis patients that interfere with fertilization or early embryo growth.

Altered Prostaglandins

Prostaglandins have undergone intensive investigation as possible mediators of endometriosis-associated infertility, with contradictory results. Willman et al. [19] demonstrated increased amounts of prostaglandins in the endometrium of endometriosis patients compared to controls. Meldrum and

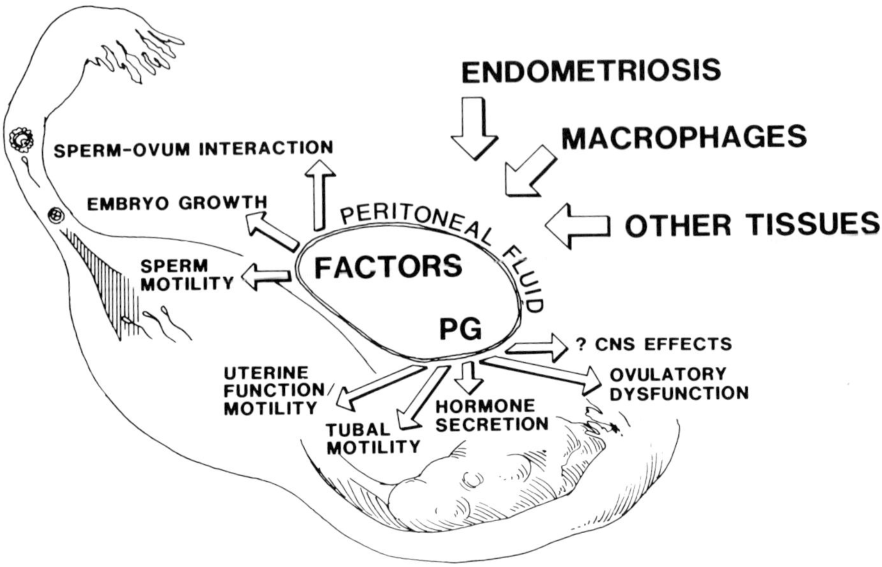

Fig. 1. Prostaglandin and peritoneal fluid alterations that may contribute to infertility in endometriosis. Prostaglandins secreted directly by implants or by "activated" macrophages may induce ovarian dysfunction or altered tubal or uterine motility. Unknown peritoneal fluid components may adversely affect sperm function, fertilization, or early embryo growth.

coworkers [20] noted that infertile patients, including those with endometriosis, had greater concentrations of prostaglandin PGF_{2a} in their peritoneal fluid than did normal women. Drake and colleagues [21,22] reported an increased peritoneal fluid volume in endometriosis patients and increased concentrations of two prostaglandin metabolites, suggesting that the total amount of prostaglandins within the pelvis of endometriosis patients was increased. They hypothesized that the prostaglandins could alter tubal motility, causing the infertility associated with endometriosis.

Vernon et al. [23] confirmed that endometriosis implants can synthesize prostaglandins and were able to demonstrate that different types of endometriosis implants had similar prostaglandin content but differed markedly in their ability to synthesize prostaglandins. The "fresh," "petechial" lesions made significantly greater amounts of prostaglandins than "burned out" implants.

Other investigators have not demonstrated a clear-cut difference in peritoneal fluid prostaglandin concentrations in women with endometriosis. Rock et al. [24] studied days 8 to 12 of the cycle and found no difference in peritoneal fluid prostaglandin levels. Badawy et al. [25] also were unable to determine differences between the two groups of patients.

On the whole, the extensive literature concerning prostaglandins in peritoneal fluid indicates that both the volume of peritoneal fluid and the concentration of prostaglandins in it are increased in infertile women with endometriosis. The prostaglandins may affect ovarian function, tubal motility, and a multitude of other functions (Fig. 1). Originally thought to come from direct secretion by the implants themselves, prostaglandin secretion from peritoneal macrophages and retrograde uterine flow may also be important sources. The finding by Vernon et al. [23] that increased secretory ability is present in the smaller lesions is potentially of great significance, explaining why minimal endometriosis may be associated with significant symptoms. In addition to prostaglandins, other secretory products may be increased as well.

IMMUNE PHENOMENA

Multiple immunologic phenomena have been put forth to explain the infertility associated with endometriosis (Fig. 2). Weed and Arquembourg [26] proposed that endometrial implants act as foreign proteins within the abdominal cavity, inciting a host immune response against the normal endometrial tissues, which in turn prevents proper nidation. To support this concept, these authors found variable degrees of fibrotic reaction and plasma cell and lymphocytic infiltrate within the endometrium of endometriosis patients, but not normal women. Immunofluorescence studies revealed that complement was present within the endometrium of most endometriosis patients, but not control women. Also, total serum complement was decreased in endometriosis patients. With conservative surgical treatment of the endometriosis, these changes were, to a degree, reversible.

Kreiner et al. [27] also studied the presence of IgG within the endometrium by immunofluorescence techniques. They confirmed that the majority of endometriosis patients (16 of 18) have antibodies present within the endometrium, whereas normal women do not; however, many subjects with histories of pelvic inflammatory disease will also stain positively with this technique. Using immunodiffusion and immunoelectrophoresis techniques, Badawy and coworkers [28] demonstrated the presence of antibodies to endometrial antigens in the serum of some endometriosis patients, but not from control women. Similarly, Wild and Shivers [29] found the presence or absence of antiendometrial antibodies in the sera of infertile women to correctly predict the diagnosis of endometriosis with approximately 70% accuracy.

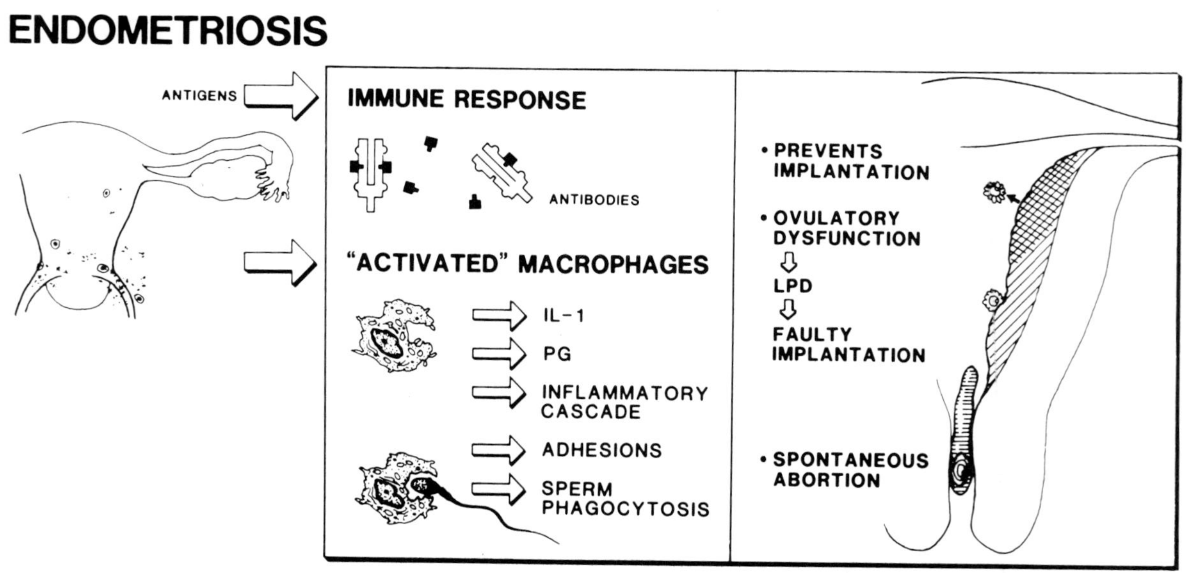
ENDOMETRIOSIS
ANTIGENS
IMMUNE RESPONSE
ANTIBODIES
"ACTIVATED" MACROPHAGES
IL-1
PG
INFLAMMATORY CASCADE
ADHESIONS
SPERM PHAGOCYTOSIS
• PREVENTS IMPLANTATION
• OVULATORY DYSFUNCTION
LPD
FAULTY IMPLANTATION
• SPONTANEOUS ABORTION

Dmowski et al. [30] investigated cell-mediated immunity in monkeys with endometriosis using injections of autologous endometrial antigens. They determined that monkeys with endometriosis had a decreased cell-mediated immunity to these antigens, despite apparent immunocompetence. In contrast, O'Shea et al. [31], using in vitro tests of human lymphocyte function, were unable to demonstrate a decreased cell-mediated immunity in endometriosis patients.

Macrophages, the primary effector arm of the immune system, have been extensively studied in endometriosis. Haney et al. [32] found women with endometriosis to have a greater concentration of macrophages in their peritoneal fluid (18.2 million/ml) compared to control women (2.6 million/ml) or infertile women without endometriosis (8.1 million/ml). Halme and coworkers [33] found no increase in peritoneal fluid concentration of these cells, but did report that increased macrophage "activation" was present.

Increased macrophage activity could decrease fertility via several mechanisms. Macrophages have been demonstrated to phagocytize and lyse sperm ascending the genital tract, especially when antisperm antibodies are present [34,35]. In testing this observation, Stone and Himsl [36] found no difference in sperm recovery at laparoscopy between endometriosis patients and other women. Macrophages are potent effectors of cell-mediated immunity and are capable of releasing many hormonal substances (such as prostaglandins and lymphokines) into the peritoneal fluid and genital tract. As mentioned previously, prostaglandins from macrophages have a wide array of possible effects on fertility.

Interleukin-1 (IL-1) is a polypeptide that is secreted by macrophages and other specialized cells as an early mediator of the immune response. Also known as "endogenous pyrogen" because it induces temperature elevation during infection, plasma concentrations of IL-1 increase during the luteal phase of the menstrual cycle in normal women [37]. IL-1 was found by Fakih et al. [38] to be increased in the peritoneal fluid of women with endometriosis, and to inhibit mouse embryo cleavage. In addition, IL-1 was also found to stimulate in vitro progesterone production from luteal cells [39].

Fig. 2. Immune abnormalities theorized to occur in endometriosis. An immune response is generated to "foreign" material in endometriosis implants. Specific antibodies to endometrial antigens are present in serum and can be detected in normal endometrium, where (along with complement and effector cells) they may cause an inflammation that prevents or impedes implantation, resulting in infertility or spontaneous abortion. Activated effector cells (macrophages and lymphocytes) aid these processes directly, phagocytize sperm, or release mediators (such as prostaglandins and interleukins) that interfere with reproduction.

Because estrogen and progesterone have been shown to increase macrophage IL-1 secretion in vitro, the possibility arises that the normal interaction between the menstrual cycle and IL-1 secretion is altered in some women with endometriosis, resulting in decreased fertility.

In summary, a large body of work concerning immune abnormalities in endometriosis has provided convincing evidence that antibodies to endometrial antigens are generated in women with endometriosis, and that other alterations in immune function are present. In particular, soluble mediators such as prostaglandins and perhaps interleukins are released into the pelvic fluid or surrounding tissues in increased amounts. In addition to affecting nidation and tubal motility, other reproductive processes may be affected. In this regard, Halme [40] has reported that macrophages may modulate corpus luteum function.

OVARIAN DYSFUNCTION

Traditionally, endometriosis has been thought to be a disease of ovulatory women; the absence of cyclic ovarian function (as in pregnancy and menopause) was associated with improvement in the disease and in fertility, which in turn led to the development of various therapies for it ("pseudomenopause," "pseudopregnancy"). Numerous lines of evidence suggest, however, that endometriosis is associated with a wide variety of abnormalities of ovarian function (Fig. 3). These phenomena could be entirely separate entities, each with its own pathophysiologic mechanism. It is important to point out, however, that they could represent varying degrees of severity of the same process — a continuum of ovarian dysfunction, which is manifested as intermittent luteal phase inadequacy when mild to complete anovulation when severe.

Anovulation

In a study of 107 infertile patients with endometriosis treated surgically, Acosta et al. [3] noted that 27% were also anovulatory. With the addition of clomiphene citrate therapy, 37% of this group became pregnant. Soules and coworkers [41] specifically investigated the incidence of ovulatory dysfunction in 350 infertile women with endometriosis; 17% were found to be either anovulatory or severely oligo-ovulatory. When both factors were treated, 43% of patients became pregnant. Using Acosta's classification, the endometriosis was mild in 39%, moderate in 59%, and severe in 2%.

Dmowski and colleagues [42] studied patients with mild endometriosis and ovulatory dysfunction. They found that maximal pregnancy rates (70%) were

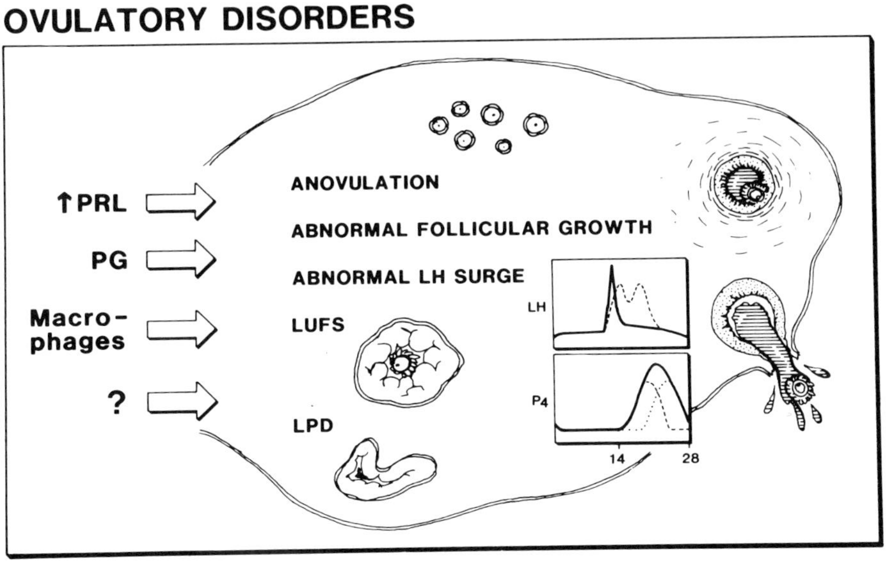

Fig. 3. Ovarian dysfunction in endometriosis. Anovulation, luteal phase defects (LPD), luteinized unruptured follicles (LUFS), abnormal luteinizing hormone surges, and excessive prolactin secretion have been associated with endometriosis. They may represent different points along a continuum of ovarian dyfunction, or be isolated phenomena causing decreased fertility.

achieved with the use of ovulatory agents following danazol therapy, when compared to ovulatory agents alone (28%).

Follicular growth may be inhibited even in women who do ovulate. Doody and colleagues [43] studied follicular development by ultrasonography in 46 infertile women with endometriosis and found a significant slowing of follicular growth rate and lengthening of time to ovulation.

The nature of this presumed endometriosis-associated ovulation defect is unknown, but it is also seen in animal models of the disease. Pittaway noted that 68% of cycles in monkeys with severe endometriosis were anovulatory [44]. In their rabbit model, Schenken and coworkers [45,46] showed that anovulation is a prime cause of endometriosis-associated infertility, and suggested that increased peritoneal fluid prostaglandins may play a causal role.

Luteal Phase Defects

No consensus exists regarding the role of luteal phase adequacy in endometriosis. Using basal body temperature charts and endometrial biopsies, Grant [47] noted that 45% of 96 patients had evidence of a luteal phase defect. Hargrove and Abraham [48] reported lower progesterone and higher estradiol levels in three pooled midluteal blood samples from women with endometriosis than in controls. After surgical therapy, Kistner [1] found 25% of his patients had evidence of luteal phase inadequacy. While examining the frequency of spontaneous abortion in endometriosis, Groll [49] noted that 56% of 80 patients demonstrated a luteal phase defect on endometrial biopsy. Cheesman et al. [50] measured urinary metabolites of progesterone in 66 infertile women daily during the luteal phase and saw a delay in the increased excretion of progesterone after ovulation in 40 patients, leading to a shortened luteal phase.

In contrast, Radwanska and Dmowski [51] found no difference from controls when midluteal levels of progesterone were examined. In a study specifically addressing this issue, Pittaway et al. [52] noted that 6 of 68 infertile women with endometriosis and 4 of 75 without the disease had luteal phase inadequacy by endometrial biopsy, fractions that are not significantly different. Finally, Saracoglu and coworkers [53] could find no difference in serum levels of estradiol and progesterone, or endometrial concentrations of their receptors, between normal women and those with endometriosis.

LUFS

The luteinized unruptured follicle syndrome (LUFS) describes the occurrence of a menstrual cycle that is ovulatory by all routine monitoring criteria (cycle length, biphasic basal body temperature, elevated luteal phase serum progesterone, secretory endometrial biopsy), but in which the oocyte remains within a follicle. The follicle fails to rupture, the ovum is entrapped, the follicle becomes luteinized, and progesterone is secreted. Techniques of diagnosing LUFS are controversial and include failure to see evidence of ovulation at laparoscopy (corpus hemorrhagicum and stigma), ultrasonic evidence of continued follicular enlargement without rupture, and failure of peritoneal fluid estradiol and progesterone levels to increase appropriately after "ovulation."

LUFS cycles were implicated as a mechanism for endometriosis-associated infertility by Brosens et al. [54], who found ovulatory stigmata at surgery in 94% of 28 control women, but only 21% of 34 infertile women with endometriosis. Subsequently, this group of investigators proposed that LUFS actually was the cause of endometriosis; they felt that LUFS prevented the high concentrations of progesterone in the follicle from entering the peritoneal fluid and retarding the implantation and growth of endometrial tissues present in the peritoneal fluid of most women at menstruation [55]. Further support linking LUFS and endometriosis comes from the monkey model of endometriosis of Schenken et al. [56], in which the primary mechanism for infertility appeared to be LUFS.

The majority of investigators, however, have not supported the concept that LUFS plays a significant, if any, role in endometriosis-associated infertility. Dmowski et al. [57] examined the ovarian surface in 199 women and could see no difference in stigma presence between endometriosis patients and other women. Kerin [58] found LUFS to be present in only 4.9% of 183 cycles when studied by ultrasound, and LUFS appeared to be a random event; a small subset of endometriosis patients had no LUFS cycles at all. Three other investigations report very little, if any, association of LUFS with endometriosis [59–61].

Abnormal LH Surge

With a variety of ovulatory dysfunctions associated with endometriosis, it is not surprising that abnormalities of the midcycle luteinizing hormone (LH) surge are being linked to the disease. Alper and Seibel [62] measured serum LH every 4 hours in 59 women around the time of the expected LH surge, and found a significantly increased rate of LH rise in the 20 endometriosis patients. Cheeseman and coworkers [63,64] have examined metabolites of luteinizing hormone, estrogen, and progesterone in daily morning urine samples, and have reported that women with endometriosis tend to have two distinct midcycle LH peaks, 2 or 3 days apart; women with more severe disease tended to have the more distinct separation. Although basal body temperature and progesterone excretion began appropriately with the first peak, the bulk of progesterone synthesis was delayed until after the second one, making the luteal phase functionally inadequate.

In a supporting case report using the monkey model of endometriosis, Schenken [65] gives a detailed account of a LUFS cycle that was carefully studied. Similar to Cheesman et al's [63,64] investigations, this report carefully documents that a LUFS cycle occurred after a blunted midcycle LH surge and after a delayed and blunted synthesis of progesterone during the luteal phase.

A defect in LH action was found by Ronnberg et al. [66], who noted a decreased content of LH receptors in follicular tissue and corpora lutea of endometriosis patients, as compared to control women.

Increased Prolactin

Inappropriate prolactin secretion has been investigated by several authors as a mechanism to explain endometriosis-associated infertility. Pathologically elevated prolactin concentrations are well known to cause infertility by inducing ovulatory disturbance (anovulation, luteal phase defects) via a hypothalamic-pituitary, and perhaps a local ovarian, effect.

Hirschowitz and coworkers [67] studied nine infertile patients with endometriosis and regular menses; eight had galactorrhea, and two had elevated prolactin levels. They termed this combination of findings the "galactorrhea-endometriosis snydrome," suggesting that galactorrhea in a woman with regular menses indicated the presence of endometriosis. Because the endometriosis, but not the galactorrhea, responded to danazol, they felt that the two were related but largely independent processes. Hargrove and Abraham [68] found that, of fourteen endometriosis patients studied for luteal phase defects, seven had galactorrhea and three had increased prolactin levels.

To examine prolactin secretion in infertile women with mild endometriosis, Muse et al. [69] studied basal and thyrotropin-releasing hormone (TRH)-stimulated prolactin concentrations in comparison to normal, fertile women. The endometriosis group had a basal concentration twice that of the fertile group, although this was not statistically significant; however, there was a significantly increased prolactin release to TRH-stimulation in the endometriosis patients, suggesting that these women may normally exhibit an excessive capacity for prolactin secretion. Gendron and coworkers [70] performed a similar study and found a higher prolactin response in normal women than in infertile women, with or without endometriosis. Radwanska et al. [71] studied prolactin concentrations during the night and found increased levels in women with endometriosis.

The normal luteal phase endometrium secretes prolactin; thinking that endometriosis implants may also secrete prolactin, possibly producing local ovarian dysfunction, Haney et al. [72] measured prolactin concentrations in the peritoneal fluid of fertile and infertile women (with or without endometriosis). They found no difference between the groups, suggesting that the implants do not secrete prolactin in sufficient quality to interfere with reproduction.

To summarize, infertile women with endometriosis have been found to have a variety of ovulation disorders. The extent to which endometriosis causes these disorders needs to be further characterized, as does the mechanism(s) involved. Whether these disorders represent individual problems, or different points along a spectrum of ovulatory dysfunction, may then be revealed.

SPONTANEOUS ABORTION

The detrimental effect of endometriosis on fertility does not end once pregnancy has been achieved. Many studies have incidentally documented an elevated spontaneous abortion rate in women with this disease; several reports have specifically addressed this issue (Table II). Among women found to have endometriosis at operation, virtually all investigators have noted that the percentage of previous pregnancies ending in spontaneous abortion was markedly elevated, generally ranging from 35% to 50% [73,74]. After conservative surgery, this rate has been uniformly observed to fall to that normally expected, approximate 15% [75,76]. Groll [49] has also noted a 7% rate after medical (danazol) therapy.

In contrast, Naples and coworkers [77] have found expectant management to be accompanied by a persistently increased risk of miscarriage. Also, in the continuing series reported by Wheeler et al. [78] and by Malinak and Wheeler [79], the preoperative spontaneous abortion rate was significantly higher in those found to have mild, compared to more severe, stages of endometriosis. Although most abortions occurred near the time of surgery, a possible source of bias in these studies, an elevated rate was present in endometriosis patients for many years prior to surgical diagnosis.

The mechanism linking endometriosis to increased risk of spontaneous abortion remains speculative. Luteal phase inadequacy is known to cause miscarriages and has been associated with endometriosis (see above). Immune dysfunction leading to faulty implantation and altered prostaglandin milieu causing aberrant ovarian, uterine, or tubal function have also been

TABLE II. Spontaneous Abortion Rates in Patients With Endometriosis and the Effect of Treatment

	Spontaneous abortion rate			
		After treatment		
References	Prior to diagnosis (%)	Expectant (%)	Conservative surgery (%)	Medical therapy (%)
Petersohn, 1970 [75]	22	—	8	—
Rock, 1981 [76]	49	—	20	—
Naples, 1981 [77]	46	—	8	—
	26	25	—	—
Olive, 1982 [73]	44	—	—	—
Groll, 1984 [49]	—	52	12	7
Pittaway, 1985 [74]	38	—	—	—
Metzger, 1986 [80]	63	19	0	—
Wheeler, 1983 [78], Malinak, 1986 [79]	37	—	9	—
Mild	49	—	9	—
Moderate	25	—	10	—
Severe	30	—	8	—

proposed. The observation that the highest spontaneous abortion rate was found in patients with mild endometriosis, when linked to the finding of Vernon et al. [23] that the "fresh" lesions of minimal endometriosis had increased prostaglandin secretory capacity, suggests that prostaglandins may play a role in this event.

Metzger et al. [80] noted pre- and postoperative spontaneous abortion rates of 63.1% and 0%, respectively, in patients treated surgically; however, women treated expectantly were discovered to have near normal postoperative rates of miscarriage (16.7% with mild disease, 21.4% with moderate). These authors suggested that untreated endometriosis does not increase the risk of spontaneous abortion and emphasized the importance of well-defined control groups in studies of this type. Other sources for bias include the preselected nature of the patients studied (compared to the general population), the inaccuracy of past medical histories, the possible therapeutic effects of surgery itself, the postoperative benefits of close medical observation and support, and the great likelihood of normal pregnancy following miscarriage.

Despite these valid concerns, endometriosis has been linked to an increased rate of spontaneous abortion by virtually all investigators. After treatment, the miscarriage rate falls to that expected, lending further support to an association between early pregnancy loss and this disease. Other causes of pregnancy wastage (ectopic pregnancy, late pregnancy loss, congenital abnormalities) have not been associated with endometriosis.

GENETIC FACTORS

Historically, endometriosis was thought to be a disease of upper-class white women: those who were also most likely to seek help for infertility. In a review of the available epidemiologic data, however, Houston was unable to find persuasive evidence linking endometriosis to a particular race or socioeconomic class [81]. A hereditary component to endometriosis was noted in companion reports by Simpson et al. [82] and Malinak et al. [83], who investigated the families of patients with the disease. They found that 6.9% of their patients' first-degree relatives (5.8% of sisters, 8.1% of mothers) were known to have endometriosis. In contrast, using the female relatives of the patients' husbands as control subjects, only 1.0% of the sisters and 0.9% of the mothers had endometriosis, a significant difference. Also, the stage of the disease tended to be more severe if other family members were affected. Although a subsequent report failed to associate endometriosis with the presence of particular HLA antigens [84], these investigations suggested that the development of endometriosis may involve a polygenic/multifactorial inheritance pattern.

This finding has several implications regarding endometriosis-associated infertility. First, women with affected relatives are at increased risk of developing the disease; they may not wish to delay childbearing unnecessarily, and an increased diagnostic suspicion should be given to symptoms that may reflect underlying endometriosis. A genetic basis for endometriosis also implies that the infertility associated with the disease also has a genetic origin (and hence a relatively discrete mechanism), and that serum or other markers for the disease could be determined in the future, revealing disease presence and progression.

COMMENT

At present, the link between endometriosis and infertility is still poorly defined. Women with severe disease (extensive adhesions and tissue destruction) have obvious anatomic obstacles causing their greatly lessened fertility, but those with seemingly trivial lesions have a smaller decrement in fertility, which is largely unexplained. Current investigation has generated evidence supporting a wide array of possible explanations: various dysfunctions of ovulation, aberrant prostaglandin metabolism, abnormal prolactin secretion, and altered immune phenomena.

Future research will determine if one, some, or none of these theories are correct. Recognizing that each proposed mechanism of infertility overlaps with the others, and that many studies looking at one mechanism also find evidence supporting other theories, Muse and Wilson [85] proposed a multivariate hypothesis in which these phenomena could all be present, to varying degrees, in women with endometriosis; this would explain the variable nature and severity of the infertility found in this disease, and many of the inconsistencies in published reports.

Currently, several clinical applications of this knowledge are possible. Female relatives of women with endometriosis should be counseled as to their increased risk of developing the disease and its sequelae. In addition to conventional diagnosis and treatment, infertile women with endometriosis should be very carefully evaluated for appropriate follicular growth and ovulation, luteal phase inadequacy, and excessive prolactin secretion. Finally, once pregnancy has been achieved, the increased risk of spontaneous abortion mandates close observation during the first trimester.

For patients in whom very thorough evaluation and treatment fails to overcome endometriosis-associated infertility, the above information provides a basis for empiric therapies. Thinking that refractory infertility may be due to a subtle ovulatory dysfunction, ovulation induction techniques, particularly after suppressive therapy, may be applied to endometriosis patients who would not normally be candidates for such therapy. Similarly, bromocryptine treatment to lower prolactin secretion, progesterone administration for luteal phase support, intrauterine insemination with "washed" semen, and in vitro fertilization and embryo transfer are potential therapies that may be appropriate for very carefully selected patients. Until further research can define the nature of endometriosis-associated infertility, and provide specific treatments for it, such empiric therapies may increase fertility and give hope to carefully counseled infertile women who have exhausted all other avenues of treatment.

REFERENCES

1. Kistner RW: Management of endometriosis in the infertile patient. Fertil Steril 26:1151, 1975.
2. Spangler DB, Jones GS, Jones HW: Infertility due to endometriosis: conservative surgical therapy. Am J Obstet Gynecol 109:850, 1971.
3. Acosta AA, Buttram VC, Besch PK, Malinak LR, Franklin RR, Vanderheyden JD: A proposed classification of pelvic endometriosis. Obstet Gynecol 42:19, 1973.
4. The American Fertility Society: Revised American Fertility Society classification of endometriosis: 1985. Fertil Steril 43:351, 1985.
5. Guzick DS, Bross DS, Rock JA: Assessing the efficacy of the American Fertility Society's classification of endometriosis: application of a dose-response methodology. Fertil Steril 38:171, 1982.
6. Olive DL, Haney AF: Endometriosis-associated infertility: a critical review of therapeutic approaches. Obstet Gynecol Surv 41:538, 1986.
7. Schenken RS, Malinak LR: Conservative surgery versus expectant management for the infertile patients with mild endometriosis. Fertil Steril 37:183, 1982.
8. Butler L, Wilson EA, Belisle S, Gibson M, Albrecht B, Schiff I, Stillman R: Collaborative study of pregnancy rates following danazol therapy of stage I endometriosis. Fertil Steril 41:373, 1984.
9. Seibel MM, Berger MJ, Weinstein FG, Taymor M: The effectiveness of danazol on subsequent fertility in minimal endometriosis. Fertil Steril 38:534, 1982.
10. Jansen RPS: Minimal endometriosis and reduced fecundability: prospective evidence from an artificial insemination by donor program. Fertil Steril 46:141, 1986.
11. Hammond MG, Jordan S, Sloan CS: Factors affecting pregnancy rates in a donor insemination program using frozen semen. Am J Obstet Gynecol 155:480, 1986.
12. Strathy JH, Molgaard CA, Coulam CB, Melton LJ: Endometriosis and infertility: a laparoscopic study of endometriosis among fertile and infertile women. Fertile Steril 38:667, 1982.
13. Morcos RN, Gibbons WE, Findley WE: Effect of peritoneal fluid on in vitro cleavage of 2-cell mouse embryos: possible role in infertility associated with endometriosis. Fertil Steril 44:678, 1985.
14. Gerrity M, Rinehart JS, Shapiro SS: The effect of human peritoneal fluid on embryonic development. Annual meeting of the American Fertility Society, 1985, Abstract #58.
15. Sueldo CE, Lambert H, Steinleitner AJ, Swanson JA: Effect of peritoneal fluid on murine sperm-ova interaction. Annual meeting of the American Fertility Society, 1986, Abstract #23.

16. Halme J, Hall JL: Effect of pelvic fluid from endometriosis patients on human sperm penetration of zona-free hamster ova. Fertil Steril 37:573, 1982.
17. Chacho KJ, Chacho MS, Andresen PJ, Scommegna A: Peritoneal fluid in patients with and without endometriosis: prostanoids and macrophages and their effect on the spermatozoa penetration assay. Am J Obstet Gynecol 154:1290, 1986.
18. Muse KN, Estes S, Vernon M, Zavos P, Wilson EA: Effect of endometriosis on sperm motility in peritoneal fluid in vitro. American Fertility Society, 1986, Abstract #286.
19. Willman EA, Collins WP, Clayton SG: Studies in the involvement of prostaglandins in uterine symptomatology and pathology. Br J Obstet Gynaecol 83:337, 1976.
20. Meldrum DR, Shamonki IM, Clark KE, Rubinstein LM, Lebherz TB: Prostaglandin content of ascitic fluid in endometriosis: a preliminary report. Annual meeting of the Pacific Coast Fertility Society, 1977.
21. Drake TS, Metz SA, Grunert GM, O'Brien WF: Peritoneal fluid volume in endometriosis. Fertil Steril 34:280, 1980.
22. Drake TS, O'Brien WF, Ramwell PW, Metz SA: Pertioneal fluid thromboxane B_2 and 6-Keto-Prostaglandin F_{1a} in endometriosis. Am J Obstet Gynecol 140:401, 1981.
23. Vernon MW, Wilson EA: Enhanced prostaglandin F production by endometriotic implants from patients with mild and moderate endometriosis. American Fertility Society, 1986, Abstract #289.
24. Rock JA, Dubin NH, Ghodgaonkar RB, et al.: Cul-de-sac fluid in women with endometriosis: fluid volume and prostanoid concentration during the proliferative phase of the cycle—days 8 to 12. Fertil Steril 37:747, 1982.
25. Badawy S, Marshall L, Gabal A, Nusbaum L: The concentrations of 13, 14-dihydro-125-keto-prostaglandin F and prostaglandin E in peritoneal fluid of patients with and without endometriosis. Fertil Steril 38:166, 1982.
26. Weed JC, Arquembourg PC: Endometriosis: can it produce an autoimmune response resulting in infertility? Clin Obstet Gynecol 23:885, 1980.
27. Kreiner D, Fromowitz FB, Richardson DA, Kenigsberg D: Endometrial immunofluorescence associated with endometriosis and pelvic inflammatory disease. Fertil Steril 46:243, 1986.
28. Badawy SZ, Cuenca V, Stitzel A, Jacobs RBD, Tomar RH: Autoimmune phenomena in patients with endometriosis. Obstet Gynecol 63:271, 1984.
29. Wild RA, Shivers CA: Antiendometrial antibodies in patients with endometriosis. Am J Reprod Immunol Microbiol 8:84, 1985.
30. Dmowski WP, Steele RW, Baker GF: Deficient cellular immunity in endometriosis. Am J Obstet Gynecol 141:377, 1981.
31. O'Shea RT, Wright A, Jones WR: Cell mediated immunity in endometriosis. Annual meeting of the American Fertility Society, 1986, Abstract #311.
32. Haney AF, Muscato JJ, Weinberg JB: Peritoneal fluid cell populations in fertility patients. Fertil Steril 35:696, 1981.
33. Halme J, Becker S, Hammond M, Raj M: Increased activation of peritoneal macrophages in infertile women with endometriosis. Annual meeting of the Society for Gynecologic Investigation, 1982, Abstract #316.
34. Muscato JJ, Haney AF, Weinberg JB: Sperm phagocytosis by human peritoneal macrophages: a possible cause of infertility in endometriosis. Am J Obstet Gynecol 144:503, 1982.
35. London SN, Haney AF, Weinberg JB: Macrophages and infertility: enhancement of human macrophage-mediated sperm killing by antisperm antibodies. Fertil Steril 43:274, 1985.

36. Stone SC, Himsl K: Peritoneal recovery of motile and nonmotile sperm in the presence of endometriosis. Fertil Steril 46:338, 1986.
37. Cannon JG, Dinarello CA: Increased plasma interleukin-1 activity in women after ovulation. Science 227:1247, 1985.
38. Fakih H, Baggett B, Holtz G, Williamson HO, Rust PF, Tsang KY, Lee JC: Interleukin-1: a possible role in infertility associated with endometriosis. Annual meeting of the American Fertility Society, 1986, Abstract #3.
39. Fakih H, Polan ML, Romero R, Mathur R, Durum S, Williamson HO: Interleukin-1 (IL-1) stimulates progesterone production from granulosa cells. Annual meeting of the American Fertility Society, 1986, Abstract #P158.
40. Halme J, Hammond MG, Syrop CH, Talbert LM: Peritoneal macrophages modulate human granulosa-luteal cell progesterone production. J Clin Endocrinol Metab 61:912, 1985.
41. Soules MR, Malinak LR, Bury R, Poindexter A: Endometriosis and anovulation: a coexisting problem in the infertile female. Am J Obstet Gynecol 125:412, 1976.
42. Dmowski WP, Radwanska E, Binor Z, Rana N: Mild endometriosis and ovulatory dysfunction: effect of danazol treatment on success of ovulation induction. Fertil Steril 46:784, 1986.
43. Doody MC, Rossavik IK, Gibbons WE: Women with endometriosis have significantly abnormal ultrasonographic follicular growth parameters. Annual meeting of the American Fertility Society, 1986, Abstract #263.
44. Pittaway DE, Klimek M, Koritnik DR: Ovulatory dysfunction in rhesus monkeys with severe endometriosis. American Fertility Society, 1986, Abstract #253.
45. Schenken RS, Asch RH: Surgical induction of endometriosis in the rabbit: effects on fertility and concentrations of peritoneal fluid prostaglandins. Fertil Steril 34:581, 1980.
46. Schenken RS, Walters MD: Ovulation and tubal ovum transport in rabbit with endometriosis. Annual meeting of the Society for Gynecologic Investigation Abstract, 1986, #361.
47. Grant A: Additional sterility factors in endometriosis. Fertil Steril 17:514, 1966.
48. Hargrove JT, Abraham GK: Abnormal luteal function in endometriosis. Fertil Steril 34:302, 1980.
49. Groll M: Endometriosis and spontaneous abortion. Fertil Steril 41:933, 1984.
50. Cheesman KL, Cheesman SD, Chatterton RT, Cohen MR: Alterations in progesterone metabolism and luteal function in infertile women with endometriosis. Fertil Steril 40:590, 1983.
51. Radwanska E, Dmowski WP: Luteal function in infertile women with endometriosis. Infertility 4:269, 1981.
52. Pittaway DE, Maxson W, Daniell J, Herbert C, Wentz AC: Luteal phase defects in infertility patients with endometriosis. Fertil Steril 39:712, 1983.
53. Saracoglu OF, Aksel S, Yeoman RR, Wiebe RH: Endometrial estradiol and progesterone receptors in patients with luteal phase defects and endometriosis. Fertil Steril 43:851, 1985.
54. Brosens IA, Konickx PR, Corveleyn PA: A study of plasma progesterone, oestradiol-17B, prolactin and LH levels, and of the luteal phase appearance of the ovaries in patients with endometriosis and infertility. Br J Obstet Gynaecol 85:246, 1978.
55. Konickx PR, Ide P, Vandenbroucke W, Brosens IA: New aspects of the pathophysiology of endometriosis and associated infertility. J Reprod Med 24:257, 1980.

56. Schenken RS, Asch RH, Williams RF, Hodgen GD: Etiology of infertility in monkeys with endometriosis: luteinized unruptured follicles, luteal phase defects, pelvic adhesions, and spontaneous abortions. Fertil Steril 41:122, 1984.
57. Dmowski WP, Rao R, Scommegna A: The luteinized unruptured follicle syndrome and endometriosis. Fertil Steril 33:30, 1980.
58. Kerin JF, kirby C, Morris D, McEvoy M, Ward B, Cox LW: Incidence of the luteinized unruptured follicle phenomenon in cycling women. Fertil Steril 40:620, 1983.
59. Holtz G, Williamson HO, Mathur RS, Landgrebe SC, Moore EE: Luteinized unruptured follicle syndrome in mild endometriosis. Assessment with biochemical parameters. J Reprod Med 30:643, 1985.
60. Dhont M, Serreyn R, Duvivier P, Vanluchene E, Boever JD, Vandekerckhove D: Ovulation stigma and concentration of progesterone and estradiol in peritoneal fluid: relation with fertility and endometriosis. Fertil Steril 41:872, 1984.
61. Donnez J, Langerock S, Thomas K: Peritoneal fluid volume, 17 beta-estradiol, and progesterone concentration in women with endometriosis and/or luteinized unruptured follicle syndrome. Gynecol obstet Invest 16:210, 1983.
62. Alper M, Seibel M: Aberrant surge of luteinizing hormone in women with endometriosis. Annual meeting of the Society for Gynecologic Investigation, 1986, Abstract #278.
63. Cheesman KL, Ben-Num I, Chatterton RT, Cohen MR: Relationship of luteinizing hormone, pregnanediol-3-glucuronide, and estriol-16-glucuronide in urine of infertile women with endometriosis. Fertil Steril 38:542, 1982.
64. Cheesman KL, Cheesman SD, Chatterton RT, Cohen MR: Alterations in progesterone metabolism and luteal function in infertile women with endometriosis. Fertil Steril 40:590, 1983.
65. Schenken RS, Werlin LB, Williams RF, Prihoda TJ, Hodgen GD: Histologic and hormonal documentation of the luteinized unruptured follicle syndrome. Am J Obstet Gynecol 154:839, 1986.
66. Ronnberg L, Kauppila A, Rajaniemi H: Luteinizing hormone receptor disorder in endometriosis. Fertil Steril 42:64, 1984.
67. Hirschowitz JS, Soler NG, Wortsman J: The galactorrhea-endometriosis syndrome. Lancet 1:896, 1978.
68. Hargrove JT, Abraham GK: Abnormal luteal function in endometriosis. Fertil Steril 34:302, 1980.
69. Muse K, Wilson EA, Jawad MJ: Prolactin hyperstimulation in response to thyrotropin-releasing hormone in patients with endometriosis. Fertil Steril 38:419, 1982.
70. Gendron R, Ainmelk Y, Belisle S: Prolactin response to thyrotropin-releasing hormone in patients with mild endometriosis. Annual meeting of the Canadian Fertility Society, 1983.
71. Radwanska E, Heig I, Rana N, Dmowski WP: Nocturnal prolactin (PRL) levels in infertile women with and without endometriosis. Annual meeting of the Society for gynecologic Investigation, 1985, Abstract #109P.
72. Haney AF, Handwerger S, Weinberg JB: Peritoneal fluid prolactin in infertile women with endometriosis: lack of evidence of secretory activity by endometrial implants. Fertil Steril 42:935, 1984.
73. Olive DL, Franklin RR, Gratkins LV: The association between endometriosis and spontaneous abortion. A retrospective clinical study. J Reprod Med 27:333, 1982.
74. Pittaway DE, Vernon C, Fayez JA: Spontaneous abortions in women with endometriosis. American Fertility Society Annual Meeting, 1985, Abstract #90.

75. Petersohn L: Fertility in patients with ovarian endometriosis before and after treatment. Acta Obstet Gynecol Scand 49:331, 1970.
76. Rock JA, Guzick DS, Sengos C, Schweditsch M, Sapp KC, Jones HW Jr: The conservative surgical treatment of endometriosis: evaluation of pregnancy success with respect to the extent of disease as categorized using contemporary classification systems. Fertil Steril 35:131, 1981.
77. Naples JD, Batt RE, Sadigh H: Spontaneous abortion rate in patients with endometriosis. Obstet Gynecol 57:509, 1981.
78. Wheeler JM, Johnston BM, Malinak LR: The relationship of endometriosis to spontaneous abortion. Fertil Steril 39:656, 1983.
79. Malinak LR, Wheeler JM: Association of endometriosis with spontaneous abortion, prognosis for pregnancy, and risk of recurrence. Semin Reprod Endocrinol 3:361, 1986.
80. Metzger DA, Olive DL, Stohs GF, Franklin RR: Association of endometriosis and spontaneous abortion: effect of control group selection. Fertil Steril 45:18, 1986.
81. Houston DE: Evidence for the risk of pelvic endometriosis by age, race, and socioeconomic status. Epidemiol Rev 6:167, 1984.
82. Simpson JL, Elias S, Malinak LR, Butram VC: Heritable aspects of endometriosis. I. Genetic studies. Am J Obstet Gynecol 137:327, 1980.
83. Malinak LR, Buttram VC, Elias S, Simpson JL: Heritable aspects endometriosis. II. Clinical characteristics of familial endometriosis. Am J Obstet Gynecol 137:332, 1980.
84. Simpson JL, Malinak LR, Elias S, Carson S, Radvany RA: HLA associations in endometriosis. Am J Obstet Gynecol 148:395, 1984.
85. Muse KN, Wilson EA: How does mild endometriosis cause infertility? Fertil Steril 38:145, 1982.

Endometriosis, pages 111–140

Chapter 7
Medical Therapy for Endometriosis

Robert L. Barbieri, M.D., and Mark D. Hornstein, M.D.

Department of Obstetrics and Gynecology, Brigham and Women's Hospital and the Laboratory of Human Reproduction and Reproductive Biology, Harvard Medical School, Boston, Massachusetts 02115

INTRODUCTION

During the past four decades, the medical management of endometriosis has become significantly more sophisticated. In the early 1950s, the high-dose estrogen regimen of Karnaky was the only available hormonal treatment for endometriosis [1]. In the 1960s and 1970s, Kistner's "pseudopregnancy" and "progestin-only" regimens dominated the medical management of endometriosis [2–4]. During the 1980s, danazol has become the primary hormonal agent used in the treatment of endometriosis [5–7]. It is likely that the 1990s will witness the ascendancy of the gonadotropin-releasing hormone (GnRH) agonists for the treatment of endometriosis [8]. These advances have significantly expanded the hormonal armamentarium of the gynecologist treating endometriosis. Proper use of these agents requires a thorough understanding of the hormonal responses of endometriotic tissues and an appreciation of the pharmacologic properties of the available agents.

HORMONAL RESPONSES OF ENDOMETRIOTIC TISSUES

The central dogma that guides the hormonal therapy of endometriosis is the belief that steroid hormones are the major regulators of growth and function of endometriotic tissue. Both clinical and laboratory observations support this central dogma. The primary role of steroid hormones in regulating the

Supported in part by NIH grant HD-18292.

growth of endometriotic implants is supported by the following clinical observations: 1) endometriosis rarely occurs prior to the menarche, 2) menopause, either surgical or natural, usually produces an improvement in preexisting endometriosis, and 3) new cases of endometriosis occur very rarely after the menopause unless exogenous estrogens are being administered.

Laboratory evidence obtained from both in vitro and in vivo experiments supports the central role of steroids in regulating the growth of endometriotic implants. Laboratory studies have demonstrated that the majority of human endometriotic implants contain estrogen receptors (ER), progesterone receptors (PR), and androgen receptors (AR) [9–11]. These findings suggest that endometriotic implants respond to all three classes of steroid hormones. Laboratory models of experimental endometriosis in the rat and rabbit indicate that estrogen stimulates the growth of endometriotic tissue [12] and androgens tend to induce atrophy in endometriotic implants. The role of progesterone in the regulation of endometriotic tissue is controversial. Progesterone alone may actually support the growth of endometriotic tissue [12]. However, the synthetic progestogens, many of which have androgenic properties, appear to inhibit the growth of endometriotic tissue.

The polarity of response of endometriotic tissue to androgens and estrogens is the Ying and Yang upon which all current hormonal therapy of endometriosis is based. Three observations complicate this simplistic conceptualization. 1) A small percentage of endometriotic implants ($\sim 5\%$) do not contain significant concentrations of either estrogen or progesterone receptors [9,11]. These lesions may be relatively resistant to hormonal therapy. 2) Microheterogeneity within endometriotic lesions may make the steroid receptor positive cell populations more susceptible to hormonal manipulations than the steroid receptor negative cell populations. 3) Some endometriotic lesions that contain progesterone receptors do not demonstrate typical functional (increased 17β-hydroxysteroid dehydrogenase enzyme activity) or structural (secretory changes) responses to progesterone stimulation [11]. This observation suggests that in some endometriotic implants the intranuclear steroid receptors are uncoupled from their site of action (DNA).

The polarity of response of endometriotic tissue to androgens and estrogens is the basis for the two hormonal strategies that are most often used to treat endometriosis. One basic strategy is to create an acyclic, low-estrogen hormonal environment. The low estrogen levels cause atrophy of the endometriotic tissues. The acyclic environment helps minimize the chance of miniature "menstruation" in the endometriotic implants and prevents reseeding of implants from the retrograde transport of normal endometriosis during menstruation. An acyclic, low-estrogen environment is best produced by bilateral oophorectomy, or with the use of GnRH-agonists (Table I). The second basic strategy is to produce a hormonal environment high in androgens or synthetic progestogens. The high-androgen environment directly produces atrophy of endometriotic implants. It is important to note that most synthetic progestogens have some androgenic properties. The high androgen/progestogen strategy also results in low, acyclic estrogen levels by interfering with ovarian follicular development. Table I summarizes these different strategies.

The schematic classification system presented in Table I (based on steroid hormone profiles) is a convenient method by which to categorize currently available hormonal regimens for the treatment of endometriosis. However, two new areas of investigation suggest that the regulation of endometriotic growth and function may be significantly more complex than currently appreciated. These new experimental findings suggest that paracrine protein growth factors and immunologic factors may regulate the development of endometriosis. Each of these new areas of research is discussed briefly.

Evidence is mounting that there is regulatory "cross-talk" between the epithelial and stromal elements of the endometrium. This regulation is mediated, in part, by "paracrine" protein growth factors secreted by the stroma that cause morphogenetic changes in the epithelium. The most dramatic examples of endometrial stromal-epithelial interactions have been the "recombination" experiments of Cunha and associates [13–15]. Cunha reported that the coculturing of vaginal stroma with endometrial epithelium caused the endometrial epithelium to keratinize and secrete mucin, just like vaginal

TABLE I. Hormonal Regimens Available for the Treatment of Endometriosis

Classification of hormonal regimens	Typical endocrine environment produced	Common unwanted effects
A) Gonadotropin-releasing hormone agonists	Acyclic, low estrogen	Vasomotor symptoms Atrophy of secondary sexual characteristics
Oophorectemy		Accelerated bone loss
B) Danazol Methyltestosterone	Acyclic, high androgen, low estrogen	Weight gain, "breakthrough bleeding", acne, oily skin, hirsutism, voice changes
C) Medroxyprogesterone acetate Gestrinone Norethindrone	Acyclic, high progestogen, low estrogen	Weight gain, bloating, depression, "breakthrough bleeding"
D) Noncyclic oral contraceptives	Acyclic, high progestogen, moderate estrogen	Nausea, "breakthrough bleeding"

epithelium. In like manner, the coculturing of endometrial stroma with vaginal epithelium caused the "squamous" vaginal epithelium to change to a simple columnar epithelium. Cunha concluded that the endometrial stroma secretes paracrine growth factor(s) that regulate epithelial function. These paracrine growth factor(s) have not yet been characterized. However, identification of proteins involved in endometrial epithelial-stromal interaction may stimulate the development of new methods for treating endometriosis.

Evidence is mounting that pelvic endometriosis is often associated with activation of the immune system. Weed [16] has hypothesized that endometriotic proteins found in the peritoneal cavity of patients with endometriosis may be recognized by the immune system as "foreign," triggering an "autoimmune" response. Evidence to support the association of endometriosis and immune activation includes: 1) increased peritoneal fluid lymphocytes, macrophages, complement, and antibodies [17,18], and 2) increased circulating antiendometrial antibodies in women with endometriosis [19]. It is conceivable that this immune activation produces an environment toxic to oocytes and embryos, resulting in infertility. In addition, the prostaglandins and lymphokines produced by the immune system may cause the pelvic pain and peritoneal scarring associated with endometriosis. It is probable that modulation of the immune system may become a method of treating endometriosis.

INDICATIONS FOR THE HORMONAL TREATMENT OF ENDOMETRIOSIS

Although endometriosis is one of the most common gynecologic diseases, few prospective, controlled clinical trials of therapeutic regimens for this disease have been completed. Current recommendations concerning the treatment of endometriosis are largely derived from clinical experience and not from controlled scientific studies. Controlled scientific studies may dramatically change our current approach to the clinical management of endometriosis. Until these scientific studies are completed, therapeutic decisions must be based on currently available clinical data, much of which are anecdotal.

Patients with endometriosis usually present with one of three complaints: 1) pelvic pain, 2) adnexal mass, or 3) infertility. Each clinical presentation requires a different therapeutic approach, and these considerations are discussed below. A few general considerations apply to all clinical presentations of endometriosis. One of these considerations is the widely accepted rule that hormonal therapy for endometriosis should never be instituted until the diagnosis of endometriosis has been confirmed by laparoscopy or laparotomy. Other major considerations governing the hormonal therapy of endometriosis are reviewed below.

Pelvic Pain

Multiple studies strongly suggest that hormonal therapy for patients with pelvic pain and endometriosis completely or partially improves the pain symptoms in approximately 90% of treated patients [5–7]. Treatment with antiprostaglandin agents, such as ibuprofen, is also often successful, and no studies are available to directly compare these two approaches. In general, women with severe endometriosis who are over 40 years of age and have completed their families are probably best treated by a definitive surgical procedure (bilateral oophorectomy and hysterectomy) [20]. Young women with endometriosis and pelvic pain can often be successfully treated with hormonal therapy.

Adnexal Mass

Most persistent, large (>6 cm) ovarian masses need to be surgically removed. Surgical removal of persistent ovarian masses is simultaneously diagnostic and therapeutic. The surgical removal of an endometrioma should be followed by the development of a long-term therapeutic plan. The majority of young women who have had an endometrioma surgically removed will have a recurrence of their endometriosis within 5 years. For young patients, long-term hormonal therapy may be necessary to prevent the repetitive recurrence of endometriomas.

Infertility

There is no strong scientific evidence to support the hypothesis that mild or moderate endometriosis causes infertility [21,22]. Given this fact, it is not surprising that there are no controlled clinical studies that demonstrate that the treatment of mild or moderate endometriosis "cures" infertility [23,24]. The use of hormonal or surgical therapy for the treatment of infertility associated with mild or moderate endometriosis is a clinical decision to be made jointly by the doctor and patient after all alternatives are explored. Severe endometriosis probably does cause infertility. In cases of infertility associated with severe endometriosis, conservative surgical therapy is usually necessary to improve the fecundity rate. In our experience, preoperative hormonal therapy makes the surgical procedure technically easier to perform [6]. This is true whether the planned operation is a cystectomy, a conservative laparotomy, or a definitive surgical procedure.

Recurrence

The only definitive therapy of endometriosis is surgical removal of both ovaries and the uterus. Patients with endometriosis who are treated with hormonal therapy or conservative surgery have a very high chance of developing recurrent endometriosis after the completion of therapy. Patients need to clearly understand that hormonal therapy of endometriosis will not result in a "cure" of the disease.

HORMONAL AGENTS AVAILABLE FOR THE TREATMENT OF ENDOMETRIOSIS

Currently, six agents dominate the hormonal therapy of endometriosis. Three of these agents, danazol, gestrinone, and gonadotropin-releasing hormone (GnRH) agonists are discussed in detail, since they are likely to be the most commonly used agents for the treatment of endometriosis during the next 15 years. Progestin-only medications, acyclic oral estrogen/progestin combinations, and methyltestosterone regimens are discussed in brief, since the use of these agents for the treatment of endometriosis is likely to decline.

Danazol

Danazol is an isoxazole derivative of the synthetic steroid 17α-ethinyltestosterone (Fig. 1). The pharmacology of danazol is exceedingly complex and is best discussed in terms of the molecular pharmacology of the drug. Current laboratory findings suggest that danazol interacts with only two major classes of human proteins: 1) steroid hormone receptors and 2) enzymes of steroidogenesis. The entire pharmacologic profile of danazol (and danazol's metabolites) can be explained by danazol's interaction with these two classes of proteins.

Metabolites of danazol. Danazol is metabolized to at least 60 different products in vivo [25]. One of the major metabolites of danazol is 17α-ethinyltestosterone [25,26]. This steroid is known to be both a progestogen

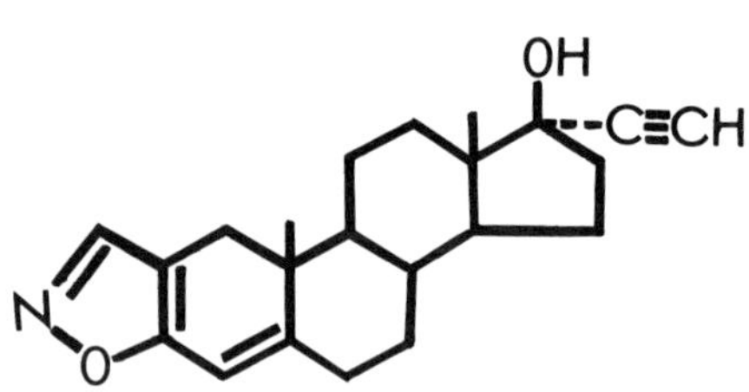

Fig. 1. The chemical structure of danazol.

and a weak androgen [27]. 17α-ethinyltestosterone is a relatively effective inhibitor of pituitary LH and FSH secretion [27]. The large number of metabolites of danazol, and the unique biological properties of some of these metabolites, complicates the pharmacology of this drug. To simplifiy the presentation, this review focuses on the pharmacologic properties of the parent compound, danazol. The reader should be aware that some of the metabolites of danazol may contribute to its therapeutic effects.

Danazol and steroid-binding proteins. Steroid hormones produce biologic effects in steroid responsive tissues by first binding to intranuclear steroid receptors. Recent evidence suggests that cytoplasmic steroid receptors are a laboratory artifact. In vivo the vast majority of cell steroid receptors are intranuclear. Via mechanisms that remain unclear, the steroid-receptor complex initiates changes in the rate of transcription of tissue-specific genes. Naturally occurring steroids demonstrate a great deal of specificity in their interaction with receptors. For example, estradiol binds well to the estradiol receptor but does not significantly interact with androgen or progesterone receptors. In sharp contrast, many synthetic steroid hormones are less specific in their receptor-binding profiles and can bind to multiple classes of receptors. In the first systematic screening of the interaction of danazol with steroid-binding proteins, our laboratory reported that danazol bound to intracellular androgen, progesterone, glucocorticoid, and estrogen receptors [28]. Subsequently, numerous other investigators have confirmed our original findings [29–34].

In addition to binding to intracellular receptors, danazol also interacts with two circulating steroid-binding proteins: sex hormone-binding globulin (SHBG) and corticosteroid-binding globulin (CBG) [35,36]. The interaction of danazol with each of these steroid-binding proteins is discussed below. Table II reviews these interactions.

The interaction of a steroid with an intracellular steroid receptor system can result in three possible outcomes. The steroid can produce the biological effects characteristic of that intracellular receptor system (agonist). Alternatively, the steroid can block the biologic effects typically seen after stimulation of the receptor system (antagonist). The final possibility is that the steroid can produce a mixed pattern of agonistic and antagonistic effects. For example, in androgen receptor bioassays (prostatic growth), danazol appears to be a potent androgen agonist [28]. As noted above, androgens induce atrophy in endometriotic implants. The androgenic effect of danazol is one of the main pharmacologic means by which this drug produces atrophy in endometriotic tissue.

Danazol has been reported to bind to intranuclear estrogen receptors [33]. However, the affinity of the danazol-estrogen receptor interaction is so weak

TABLE II. Interaction of Danazol With Intracellular Androgen, Progesterone, Estrogen, Glucocorticoid Receptors and With Circulating Steroid-binding Proteins

	Dissociation constant (K_i) for danazol binding to receptor (M)	Danazol biologic activity
Receptor system		
Androgen	10^{-9}	Agonist
Progestin	10^{-8}	Mixed agonist-antagonist
Glucocorticoid	10^{-7}	Agonist
Estrogen	10^{-5}	No significant biologic effects
Steroid-binding proteins		
SHBG	10^{-8}	Causes large increase in free testosterone
CBG	10^{-7}	Causes small increase in free cortisol

that we do not believe this interaction has any clinical significance [28]. Danazol interacts with glucocorticoid receptors, and preliminary evidence suggests that it is a glucocorticoid agonist [28].

Danazol binds to intranuclear progesterone receptors, but its effects in bioassays for progesterone are exceedingly complex. In some bioassays, danazol induces secretory changes in the endometrium [37–39]. This would suggest that danazol is a progesterone agonist. However, in other systems, danazol is able to block the effect of progesterone in the Clauberg assay (test substance given to estrogen-primed immature rabbits and endometrial histologic studies performed to assess progestational changes) [40]. This finding suggests that danazol is antiprogestational. Given these diverse bioassay findings, it may be best to classify danazol as a mixed agonist-antagonist with respect to the progesterone receptor system.

In summary, danazol is an androgen and glucocorticoid agonist, and a mixed agonist-antagonistic with respect to the progesterone receptor system. Danazol's poor binding to estrogen receptors suggests that it has no direct effects in this receptor system. Steroid receptors regulate cell function in a large number of diverse tissues. The effects of danazol on cell function in a variety of steroid receptor-containing tissues is briefly reviewed below.

Hypothalamus-Pituitary

By acting as an androgen agonist, danazol decreases LH and FSH secretion in castrate animals. One of danazol's main metabolites, ethinyltestosterone also suppresses LH and FSH secretion in castrate animals by acting as a progesterone agonist [27]. Although danazol suppresses LH and FSH in castrate animals, the effects of danazol on LH and FSH in animals with intact gonads is complex. The weight of evidence suggests that in women with ovaries, danazol administration does not produce a significant decrease in serum LH or FSH. This can be explained by the fact that danazol exerts a mild suppressive effect on pituitary secretion of LH and FSH, but simultaneously causes a decrease in circulating estradiol (by direct actions on the ovary), which stimulates a rise in LH and FSH. The overall effect is that danazol does not produce any significant change in serum LH or FSH.

Endometrium and Endometriotic Tissue

Danazol's androgenic properties directly suppress growth of endometrial and endometriotic tissues. Danazol's lack of estrogenic effects facilitates the androgen-mediated inhibition of growth.

Ovarian Follicle

The developing ovarian follicle appears to contain intranuclear estrogen, progesterone, and androgen receptors. The functional role of these receptors has not yet been fully characterized. However, stimulation of granulosa cell androgen receptors appears to cause an increase in progesterone production by these cells. Danazol may be able to alter normal follicular growth by interacting with these receptor systems.

Central Metabolism

Danazol's androgenic properties probably contribute to the decreased HDL cholesterol levels observed in women receiving danazol [41–43]. The atherogenic risk caused by this decrease in HDL-cholesterol remains to be fully quantitated. Danazol's androgenic and mixed progestational effects probably contribute to the mild increase in insulin resistance observed in women receiving this drug. [44].

Liver Proteins

Danazol's androgenic properties play a major role in altering the production rates of a large number of liver proteins [45]. Danazol increases the production of the following liver proteins: prealbumin, C1-esterase inhibitor, haptoglobin, transferrin, antithrombin III, prothrombin, and plasminogen. Danazol decreases the production of these liver proteins: sex hormone-binding globulin, thyroxine-binding globulin, and pregnancy zone protein.

Immune System

Substantial evidence is accumulating that steroid hormones play a major role in the regulation of the immune system. Glucocorticoid and progestogenic agonists appear to be the most important steroid regulators of the immune system. Danazol, a drug known to interact with both progesterone and glucocorticoid receptors, has been reported to be effective in the treatment of idiopathic thrombocytopenia [46] and systemic lupus erythematosis [47]. Danazol may influence the immune mechanisms involved in the development of endometriosis.

In addition to binding to intracellular steroid receptors, danazol also interacts with circulating steroid hormone-binding globulins. Danazol can displace testosterone from sex-hormone binding globulin and cortisol from corticosteroid-binding [48,49]. Of these two interactions, the danzol-induced increase in the percentage of "bioavailable testosterone" is the most important. In normal women, 40% of testosterone is bioavailable (nonSHBG bound) [50]. In women taking danazol, 80% or more of the circulating testosterone is bioavailable [50]. Therefore, part of the androgenic properties of danazol in the human may be due to the dramatic increase in bioavailable androgens caused by danazol. In addition, the observation that danazol can bind to circulating steroid-binding proteins significantly complicates the interpretation of serum total steroid concentrations in patients receiving this drug.

Danazol and enzymes of steroidogenesis. In 1977, our laboratory was the first to report that danazol inhibited multiple enzymes of steroidogenesis [51–53]. We observed that concentrations of danazol similar to those in the circulation of women taking 800 mg per day of the drug (2 μM) inhibited multiple enzymes involved in ovarian, testicular, and adrenal steroidogenesis. These enzymes included: 1) 3β-hydroxysteroid dehydrogenase isomerase, 2) 17α-hydroxylase, 17-20-lyase complex, 3) 17β-hydroxysteroid dehydrogenase, 4) 11β-hydroxylase, and 5) 21-hydroxylase [51–53]. The clinical importance of these in vitro findings is still being investigated.

Five studies suggest that danazol may directly inhibit steroidogenesis in vivo. Asch and associates [54] demonstrated that danazol shortens the luteal phase and decreases progesterone production in intact monkeys via a direct effect on the ovary. In the critical experiment, danazol was administered to monkeys starting with the first postovulatory day. Compared with control animals, danazol-treated monkeys did not respond to exogenously administered hCG with a normal rise in progesterone production. This suggests that danazol directly inhibited steroidogenesis in the monkey corpus luteum. Wentz and Sapp [55] have reported data that suggest a similar phenomenon may occur in humans.

Steingold and colleagues [56] have reported data suggesting that danazol blocks the normal estrogen rise usually seen in women receiving exogenously administered human menopausal gonadotropins (hMG). The estradiol rise caused by the administration of hMG was compared in five normal women treated with danazol and five normal women not treated with danazol. Danazol treatment resulted in a 50% decrease in serum estradiol. This suggests that danazol inhibited the effects of exogenous gonadotropins by a direct action on the ovary. These investigators also provided evidence that danazol is an inhibitor of the ovarian 17α-hydroxylase enzyme in vivo. All the experimental subjects were given dexamethasone. The purpose of this manipulation was to enusre that all serum C-21 and C-19 steroids were derived from the ovary. Half the subjects were then treated with danazol. In the women treated with danazol a significant increase in serum pregnenolone was observed with a concomitant decrease in serum 17-hydroxypregnenolone, androstenedione, and dehydroepiandrosterone.

Stillman and associates [57] observed that danazol may partially inhibit human adrenal 3β-hydroxysteroid dehydrogenase and 11β-hydroxylase in vivo. They measured the effect of danazol on the serum concentration of various steroids before and after ACTH stimulation. Five normally menstruating women were studied on the sixth day of two consecutive menstrual cycles; once as a pretreatment control and again after the administration of danazol, 600 mg orally per day for 6 days. Danazol administration resulted in no significant change in baseline cortisol concentration, but resulted in a significant increase in progesterone, dehydroepiandrosterone, and androstenedione concentrations. The administration of ACTH during the danazol treatment period resulted in greater increments in pregnenolone and 11-deoxycortisol and smaller increments in progesterone and cortisol than those seen in the control period. These findings suggest that danazol produces a partial inhibition of 3β-hydroxysteroid dehydrogenase and 11β-hydroxylase in vivo.

Castro-Magana and associates [58] reported a case of a female infant exposed to danazol in utero who was born with female pseudohermaphroditism and adrenal hyperplasia. In response to an ACTH challenge, the infant had a subnormal rise in cortisol, and an exaggerated rise in 17-hydroxyprogesterone and deoxycorticosterone. The abnormalities in adrenal steroidogenesis resolved "spontaneously" in the first year of life. These investigators concluded that danazol induced a block in adrenal 21- and 11β-hydroxylases, which resolved after the cessation of the exposure to danazol. Reyniak and Gurpide [59] have reported that danazol decreased gonadal testosterone production in three sisters with testicular feminization by a direct action on the gonad. In summary, substantial evidence suggests that danazol is a potent inhibitor of steroidogenesis, in vitro and in vivo.

How does danazol work? As noted above, an acyclic, high-androgen, low-estrogen environment is extremely hostile to the growth of endometriotic tissue. Danazol produces a high-androgen environment because: 1) danazol is inherently androgenic, and 2) danazol produces high levels of bioavailable testosterone by displacing this steroid from SHBG. A high-androgen environment directly inhibits the growth of endometriotic tissue. Danazol produces a low-estrogen environment by: 1) inhibiting follicular growth by "decreasing" GnRH, LH, and FSH secretion, and 2) by inhibiting follicular estrogen via a direct action on follicular steroidogenesis. The low-estrogen, high-androgen environment created by danazol is hostile to the growth of endometriotic tissue. In addition, the acyclic endocrine environment produced by danazol minimizes the chance of menstruation. This prevents the "reseeding" of the peritoneum with new implants of the retrograde transported endometrium. The acyclic endocrine environment may also decrease pelvic pain by inhibiting bleeding in the endometriotic implants.

The clinical use of danazol. Danazol should be initiated after the completion of a normal menses. It is important that danazol not be administered to a pregnant woman. Female pseudohermaphroditism is common in female offspring of mothers treated with danazol during the first and second trimesters [58,60–64]. Danazol is an effective contraceptive agent (<1% incidence of ovulation), at doses of 400 mg to 800 mg per day. However, patients with poor medication compliance can become pregnant on these doses of danazol because they are taking the drug in an intermittent fashion. Pregnancy testing and careful uterine examinations during danazol therapy will ensure the early detection of an unintended pregnancy. At doses of danazol below 400 mg per day, the incidence of ovulation is substantial. A barrier contraceptive should be used by all patients using doses of danazol below 400 mg per day. Women taking more than 400 mg per day of danazol should use a barrier contraceptive if their medication compliance is poor.

Danazol in doses of 200 mg per day or greater produces pain relief in the majority (>90%) of patients with endometriosis [65,66]. However, danazol at doses of 400 mg per day or greater is required to reliably produce amenorrhea [65,66]. Due to cost considerations, we start patients with mild or moderate endometriosis on 400 mg per day of danazol. Patients with severe endometriosis should probably be given 800 mg per day. Alternatively, some clinicians prefer to use 800 mg per day in all patients to assure maximal effect.

Cessation of menses and serum estradiol levels are good clinical and laboratory monitors of danazol therapy. Many experienced clinicians believe that the maximal therapeutic effect of danazol occurs if menses are completely suppressed. The greater the degree of estrogen suppression, the greater the likelihood that amenorrhea will occur. The interval between drug administration appears to play an important role in determining the degree of estrogen suppression [67]. For example, in one study, the mean serum estradiol concentration was 40% lower in patients receiving 200 mg of danazol every 6 hours than in patients receiving 400 mg of danazol every 12 hours [67].

Initial trials investigating the efficacy of danazol evaluated 6-month therapy regimens. This therapy interval need not be rigidly followed. Individualization of care is important when danazol is used to treat endometriosis. For example, in the patient with advanced endometriosis who is scheduled for conservative laparotomy, a 12-week preoperative course of danazol might be appropriate. For the patient with painful endometriosis who does not desire fertility and who is adamantly opposed to surgery, a 52-to 78-week course of danazol is reasonable if side effects are carefully monitored.

A concept that we have repeatedly emphasized is that danazol therapy can have major side effects [6]. As many as 85% of patients taking danazol have side effects, including androgenic changes such as acne, hirsutism, oily skin, and deepening of the voice. The voice changes can be demonstrated by acoustic analysis [68] and can persist after discontinuation of the drug [69].

As noted above, increased low-density lipoprotein cholesterol (LDL-C) and decreased high-density lipoprotein cholesterol (HDL-C) have been associated with danazol therapy [41–43]. These changes are of concern because increased LDL-C and decreased HDL-C may be associated with atherogenic changes. In patients treated with danazol, decreased thyroid-binding globulin and an associated decrease in total thyroxine have been reported [70,71], but free thyroxine and thyroid-stimulating hormone are normal. This indicates that overall thyroid gland function is not significantly altered by danazol.

One of the most frequent problems with danazol therapy is weight gain and edema (55% of treated patients). The cause(s) of these changes is unclear. Patients with hypertension can develop increased blood pressure during danazol therapy [72]. Unusual side effects of danazol include alopecia [73] and skin rashes. In patients taking warfarin, danazol has been reported to increase prothrombin time [74].

Pregnancy and breast-feeding are absolute contraindications to the use of danazol. Danazol, like other synthetic androgens, has been reported to produce mild hepatocellular damage in some patients (elevated serum glutamic oxaloacetic transaminase and serum glutamic pyruvic transaminase) [75]. Therefore, danazol is relatively contraindicated in patients with hepatic dysfunction. Since danazol can induce marked fluid retention, patients with severe hypertension, congestive heart failure, or borderline renal function may experience deterioration of their medical condition after danazol is initated.

Danazol relieves pain in 90% of patients [5–7]. The overall pregnancy rate after danazol is 37%. Patients with mild and moderate disease have pregnancy rates of 28–60% [24], which may not differ from overall rates reported with expectant therapy (50%) [23,24]. No systematic study assessing the effect of danazol on endometriomas had been reported. In general, endometriomas should be surgically removed. Clinical experience suggests that danazol can often reduce the size of endometriomas, but that it is unusual for danazol to cause complete regression of an endometrioma.

For the majority of patients with endometriosis involving organs outside the pelvis, total abdominal hysterectomy and bilateral oophorectomy are necessary; however, certain patients will refuse surgery and others are extremely poor operative risks. In these patients, danazol therapy is an alternative of last resort. Danazol has been successful in the treatment of pulmonary endometriosis [76], bowel obstruction, and ureteral obstruction [77,78] caused by endometriosis. However, once the danazol is discontinued the lesions rapidly recur.

Recurrence rates after danazol therapy for endometriosis. A major problem in the treatment of endometriosis is that the disease tends to recur unless definitive surgical therapy is performed. Following a course of danazol therapy the recurrence of symptoms and physical findings is approximately 5% to 20% per year [5,6,79–83]. A second course of danazol therapy is often successful in inducing a remission of disease symptoms and physical findings. The high recurrence rate after hormonal therapy of endometriosis should be clearly understood by patients electing this form of therapy.

Breakthrough bleeding is one of the most irritating side effects of danazol therapy. Endometrial sampling of patients with danazol-induced breakthrough bleeding usually reveals atrophic endometrium [84]. In our experience estrogen therapy usually fails to stop the bleeding. However, the use of ethinyl estradiol (0.02 mg po qD for 5 days) is probably worth considering for these patients. Danazol, at a dose of 200 mg every 6 hours, provides the greatest chance of halting the bleeding. If this is not successful, cessation of therapy by the patient is a common end point.

Currently, danazol is the most effective agent approved by the U.S. Food and Drug Administration for the treatment of endometriosis. Until the GnRH-agonists and gestrinone are approved for use, danazol will retain its premier position.

Gestrinone

Gestrinone (R2323), 13β-ethyl-17β-hydroxy-18,19 dinorpregna-4,9,11-trien-20-yn-3-one, is a 19-nortestosterone derivative manufactured by Hoechst-Roussel-Uclaf (Paris, France). It was originally developed in the 1970s as a "once-a-week" contraceptive and underwent successful trials in the United States [85], Haiti [86], and Chile [87]. It was also tried as a contraceptive implant in Brazil [88]. Its efficacy proved equivalent to already established contraceptives. Therefore, its development was abandoned during Phase II trials due to high projected developmental costs. In the 1980s, it was resurrected as a possible therapy for the medical management of endometriosis.

In vitro and in vivo studies demonstrated gestrinone to be a progesterone agonist-antagonist and an androgen agonist in rat endometrial and prostate systems [89,90]. The drug weakly binds to endometrial estrogen receptors, but it behaves as antiestrogen in vivo, perhaps due to its interaction with progestin and androgen receptors [89,90]. Human hormonally responsive cell lines confirm gestrinone's progesterone agonist-antagonist activity [91]. Gestrinone binds with high affinity to sex hormone-binding globulin, thereby increasing the percent free testosterone. The absolute concentration of free testosterone does not change due to a decrease in total testosterone [92]. Gestrinone does not inhibit steroidogenesis up to concentrations 1,000-fold greater than that utilized clinically. Additionally, gestrinone does not inhibit prostaglandin synthesis [93].

Centrally, gestrinone acts on the hypothalamic-pituitary system to suppress midcycle surges of LH and FSH. Gestrinone blocks follicular development, thus diminishing estrogen synthesis [89,91]. It may accomplish this by reducing pituitary sensitivity to GnRH [89,94].

Thus a variety of studies demonstrate gestrinone's potential usefulness as a treatment for endometriosis. Its effects are both central and peripheral. By suppressing LH and FSH secretion, it diminishes estrogen synthesis by the ovary. Additionally, it interacts with progesterone and androgen receptors to produce endometrial atrophy. The end result is an acyclic hormonal environment and atrophy of endometrial tissue with regression of endometriosis.

The clinical efficacy of gestrinone for the treatment of endometriosis has been demonstrated in several studies. A variety of doses and regimens have been tried, all confirming the drug's beneficial effects. A French study randomized patients with laparoscopy- or laparotomy-proven endometriosis to a twice-a-week or three-times-a-week regimen with 2.5 mg of gestrinone orally. Both regimens resulted in amenorrhea in 85–90% of patients with corresponding pain relief after 2 months of therapy [89]. A German study, comparing several doses of gestrinone with 600 mg/day of danazol, yielded similar symptomatic relief. Gestrinone's side effects increased at higher doses (5 mg twice a week or 2.5 mg three times a week). However, recurrence of symptoms was higher in the low-dose group, 2.5 mg twice a week [95]. Similarly impressive results were obtained in a Brazilian study that showed 95% of laparoscopy-proven endometriosis patients to be symptom-free on gestrinone 5 mg twice a week. All patients were amenorrheic by the end of the second month [96]. Although good clinical responses have been obtained on several drug schedules, an increased incidence of breakthrough ovulation occurs on lower doses. Five of ten patients on 2.5 mg/week and four of ten patients taking 5.0 mg/week were ovulatory by LH surge [97]. A 10-mg weekly dosage reduced ovulatory frequency to only 3 of 17 cycles [98].

Side effects have been generally well tolerated and similar to those of danazol. The most frequently reported side effects are acne, increased appetite, and vaginal discharge [85]. In a trial in the United States, approximately 17% of patients discontinued gestrinone because of headaches or an unacceptable bleeding pattern [85]. Other reported side effects include spotting, seborrhea, hoarseness, reduction in breast size, transient leg pain and edema, nausea, weight gain, hirsutism, depression, lightheadedness, rash, superficial phlebitis, and chloasma. The incidence of these complaints increases with length of use. When used as an oral contraceptive, greater than 50% of patients continue the drug beyond 1 year [87].

Lipid profiles in patients using gestrinone have not been well studied. However, weekly doses of gestrinone do not alter plasma cholesterol or triglyceride levels [99,100]. Effects on bone density have not been evaluated, but clinical studies of gestrinone underway in the United States will investigate this effect. Prospective randomized trials of gestrinone and danazol are currently being conducted in the United Kingdom.

Critical to the use of any agent in the treatment of endometriosis is the rapid return of menses and demonstrated fertility of patients following discontinuation of the drug. Average time for return of menses was 24 days in patients treated with 2.5 mg twice weekly and 38 days in patients treated three times weekly with 2.5 mg [89]. One patient, with a prior history of amenorrhea, failed to menstruate for 18 months after completing a course of gestrinone [100]. Overall fertility rates posttherapy have ranged from 59% to 79% [89,96,100]. However, only 23% of patients conceived if factors other than endometriosis were also present [89]. These conception rates are similar to those in patients treated with danazol. No congenital anomalies have been reported in infants conceived while their mothers were on gestrinone [85].

Gonadotropin-Releasing Hormone-Agonists (GnRH-a)

The pulsatile pattern of endogenous gonadotropin-releasing hormone (GnRH) secretion governs the production and secretion of pituitary gonadotropin. In primates, pulses of GnRH in the range of one pulse per hour are associated with normal patterns of LH and FSH secretion. Administration of GnRH at a high pulse rate (>3 pulses per hour), or in a continuous fashion, produces an initial increase in LH and FSH secretion, which is paradoxically followed by a drastic decrease in LH and FSH. This may be due to down regulation of pituitary GnRH receptor [101,102]. Therefore, continuous administration of GnRH produces a profound hypogonadotropic effect. The effect of this desensitization is to produce a hypoestrogenic environment, beneficial in the treatment of endometriosis, polycystic ovarian diseases, precocious puberty, endometrial hyperplasia, premenstrual syndrome, and uterine fibroids. GnRH analogs have also been proposed for contraception and are currently used in the treatment of prostate cancer [103]. The short half-life of naturally occurring GnRH makes it unsuitable for therapeutic applications. However, substitutions for glycine at position 6, proline at position 9, and substitution at the carboxy terminal end of the molecule have produced GnRH agonists with prolonged half-life and increased potency. Their activity appears to be related to increased binding to receptors and decreased degradation rates. All commercially available GnRH agonists contain modification at these sites [104]. A number of these agents are already available and several others are under development (see Table III) [101]. In general, all forms of GnRH agonists may be delivered by intranasal or subcutaneous routes. A long-acting depo-GnRH agonist is undergoing clinical trials as well.

Animal experiments suggest that ablation of ovarian estrogen synthesis can effectively treat endometriosis. A GnRH-agonist leuprolide, (D-Leu^6, Pro^9

TABLE III. GnRH-Agonists Currently in Clinical Trials for the Treatment of Endometriosis[a]

Structure	Name	Company/Sponsor
(D-Ser (tBu)^6, Pro^9 NEt) GnRH	Buserelin	Hoechst
(D-LEU^6, Pro^9 NEt) GnRH	Leuprolide	TAP/Abott
(D-Trp^6, NMe Leu^7, Pro^9 NEt) GnRH	Lutrelin	Wyeth
(D-Nal(2)^6) GnRH	Nafarelin	Syntex
(D-Ser (tBu)^6, Aza-Gly^{10}) GnRH	Zoladex	ICI Ltd.
(D-Trp^6, Pro^9 NEt) GnRH		Salk Institute

[a]Modified from Ref. [101].

NEt)-GnRH induced regression of surgically placed endometrial implants in monkeys despite submaximal suppression of serum estradiol. Fertility was enhanced following the cessation of therapy [105]. A similar reduction in implants was noted using Leutrelin (D-Trp^6NMe Leu^7 Pro^9 NEt) GnRH in rats [106].

Several human trials have demonstrated the efficacy of GnRH agonists in treating endometriosis. Daily 100 μg subcutaneous injection of (D-Trp^6 Pro^9-NEt)-GnRH initially led to increased estradiol concentrations in response to elevated LH. However, this was followed by castrate levels of estradiol and androgen within 10 weeks of initiation of therapy [102]. This regimen relieved symptoms of endometriosis within 1 month in all five patients tested. However, visual confirmation of regression of disease was not demonstrated [102]. The exact mechanism of pituitary desensitization is complex, but may involve a postreceptor interaction with the cellular Golgi apparatus [107,108].

A second GnRH agonist, buserelin (D-Ser $(tBu)^6$ Pro^9 NEt)-GnRH has undergone more extensive trials using both subcutaneous and intranasal dosage. An initial report using buserelin, 300 μg intranasally reduced symptoms and diminished ectopic endometriotic tissue on follow-up laparoscopy [109]. Subcutaneous therapy using buserelin 200 μg twice a day for 5 days, followed by 400 μg intranasally three times daily relieved symptoms in six of nine patients treated. All nine patients completing their therapy demonstrated improvement on follow-up laparoscopy; however, one patient had rapid recurrence of symptoms following treatment [110]. Intranasal administration of buserelin (200 μg twice daily) produced symptomatic and objective improvement in three patients including one who had failed danazol therapy [111]. In a similar trial, five patients improved on intranasal buserelin (200 μg twice daily); however, one patient's symptoms remained refractory on doses of 400 μg three times a day [112].

Another GnRH agonist, nafarelin, (D-$Nal(2)^6$) GnRH, given 500 μg intranasally twice daily for 6 months produced symptomatic relief in eight patients treated. Follow-up laparoscopy performed on seven of the patients revealed complete resolution in five, good response in one, and only a small diminution in the size of an ovarian endometrioma in another patient [113]. Several investigators have noted regression of endometriosis and relief of symptoms using doses of GnRH agonist that do not suppress estradiol to castrate levels [110,112,113]. Administration of the GnRH agonist on day 5 of the menstrual cycle increases transient elevations of estradiol, probably due to stimulation of maturing follicles in the early follicular phase. This can be virtually eliminated by starting therapy on day 2 [114]. Initiating treatment during midluteal phase completely abolishes follicular activity in monkeys by blocking recruitment of follicles [115] and may prove beneficial in humans.

The side effects of GnRH therapy are largely those of hypoestrogenemia. A major complaint has been the development of hot flashes, frequently alleviated by decreasing the dose of the GnRH agonist [113]. Treatment of menopausal women with medroxyprogesterone acetate has been shown to decrease menopausal symptoms [116]. It could be used in combination with GnRH-agonists for symptomatic relief in such patients [103]. Other menopausal symptoms reported include insomia, vaginal dryness, mild transient depression, decreased libido, and occasional breast tenderness. A single patient developed leukocytosis while on nafarelin, but leukocyte levels returned to normal following discontinuation of the medication [113]. Long-term effects on bone density and lipid metabolism have not yet been assessed. However, nafarelin decreased bone density in five of the five patients treated for leiomyomas over a 6-month period. None had bone densities fall below the normal range [117]. Menstrual function returns to normal after GnRH agonist therapy. In patients treated for endometriosis, menses generally return within 4 to 7 weeks and in all cases within 97 days. The effects of GnRH-agonists on future fertility are not well documented. In one study, one of three previously infertile patients conceived within 6 months of stopping the drug [110].

The place of GnRH agonists in the treatment of endometriosis remains speculative. They are unlikely to replace surgery for severe endometriosis and, to date, ovarian endometriomas have failed to respond to GnRH agonists [118]. Intranasal dosage has proven acceptable, but higher doses are needed than with subcutaneous delivery. Side effects have been minor and generally well tolerated. In addition, the ultimate cost may be lower to the patient than with danazol therapy. Additionally, GnRH antagonists are in development and may be potentially useful in the treatment of endometriosis, especially since they do not stimulate the ovaries [118].

Pseudopregnancy

The use of a combined estrogen-progestogen oral contraceptive in a continuous fashion for the treatment of endometriosis is often called a "pseudopregnancy" regimen [3]. Pseudopregnancy regimens result in an anovulatory-acyclic hormone environment. During pseudopregnancy treatment the endometrium often becomes inactive and frequently demonstrates changes of pseudodecidualization. Pseudopregnancy regimens produce an acyclic hormone environment, but they do expose the endometriotic lesions to significant amounts of estrogen. Although most synthetic progestins have androgenic and antiestrogenic effects, it is conceivable that in some patients the administered estrogen actually stimulates metabolic activity in the endometriotic lesions. Use of an agent with a low estrogen dose and a potent, androgenic progestogen (such as norgestrel) probably maximizes therapeutic efficacy. A standard regimen could employ 0.03 mg of ethinyl estradiol with 0.3 mg of norgestrel daily. When breakthrough bleeding occurs, the dose could be increased to 0.05 mg of ethinyl estradiol with 0.5 mg of norgestrel daily. With the next episode of breakthrough bleeding, the dose could be increased to 0.08 mg of ethinyl estradiol with 0.8 mg of norgestrel daily.

The results of one small, prospective, randomized trial of danazol versus mestranol/norethynodrel in the treatment of endometriosis demonstrates some of the problems that can be encountered with the use of a pseudopregnancy regimen [119]. Only 30% of the pseudopregnancy group reported symptomatic improvement. Some patients in the pseudopregnancy group experienced an acute increase in the severity of their symptoms. Only 18% of the patients in the pseudopregnancy group had objective evidence of improvement in their disease. Forty-one percent of the pseudopregnancy group discontinued their therapy because of side effects such as nausea, vomiting, pelvic pain, and uterine bleeding. In contrast, in the danazol group, 86% of the patients reported an improvement in symptoms, and 84% had objective improvement. The clinical impression of those who had used danazol extensively is that it is more effective than pseudopregnancy in the treatment of endometriosis.

Methyltestosterone

Methyltestosterone therapy for endometriosis has been utilized at some centers [120–122]. The usual dose is 5 mg or 10 mg linquets administered buccally every day. The therapy usually does not inhibit ovulation. Therapeutic efficacy is probably achieved via a direct androgenic effect on the endometriotic implants. Methyltestosterone provides effective relief from the symptoms of endometriosis but fertility rates after methyltestosterone have been reported to be lower than those typically seen after danazol therapy [120]. However, the validity of comparing fertility rates between different uncontrolled studies is questionable. Many physicians are reluctant to administer methyltestosterone because of the androgenic side effects experienced by the patient and because of the possibility of inadvertently continuing drug therapy while the patient is pregnant.

Progestin-Only Regimens

Numerous progestins (medroxyprogesterone acetate, norethindrone acetate, norgestrel acetate, lynestrenol) have been used as single agents for the treatment of endometriosis [2,123,124]. In general, these agents produce a hypoestrogenic-acyclic hormonal environment by suppressing ovarian follicular activity via inhibition of LH and FSH secretion. In addition, these agents may have direct effects on endometriotic tissue androgen and progesterone receptors. As noted above, many synthetic progestins are weak androgen agonists.

A major problem with the use of progestins as single agents is that large doses must be given to produce an acyclic-hypoestrogenic environment. These high doses are often associated with side effects such as bloating, weight gain, depression, and irregular uterine bleeding. Parenteral administration of large doses of medroxyprogesterone acetate in depot form is quite effective in the treatment of endometriosis (dose range, 150 mg every 3 months to 150 mg every month). This drug is *not* recommended as a first-line agent, however, because it can produce prolonged amenorrhea after termination of therapy, and the long-term safety of the agent is still controversial. Oral administration of medroxyprogesterone acetate can be effective, but large doses are required (30 to 50 mg per day [124]).

MONITORING ENDOMETRIOSIS WITH SERUM CA-125 MEASUREMENTS

During the medical therapy of endometriosis, most clinicians use the patient's symptoms and the physical examination to monitor treatment outcome. In our experience, a decrease in pelvic pain, resolution of uterosacral ligament nodularity, and a decrease in cul-de-sac induration correlate well with laparoscopically documented improvement in the endometriosis. We have recently reported that immunoassay of serum CA-125 may be a useful laboratory marker of endometriosis disease activity [125,126].

OC-125 is an IgGl monoclonal antibody that has been obtained by somatic hybridization of spleen cells from mice immunized with cells from an epithelial ovarian carcinoma cell line [127]. The antigenic determinant defined by this antibody has been designated CA-125. CA-125 is associated with a high molecular weight (>200,000 daltons) glycoprotein that is expressed on some derivatives of the coelomic epithelium [128,130]. In adults, immunocytochemical techniques have demonstrated the presence of CA-125 on the epithelium of the fallopian tube, endometrium, and endocervix and on the peritoneum, pleura, and pericardium [128,130].

An immunoradiometric assay has been developed to detect CA-125 in peripheral blood [131]. Based on the results of this assay, 82% of patients with ovarian carcinoma, but only <1% of apparently healthy controls, have elevated peripheral blood levels of CA-125 [131]. Because endometriotic lesions are likely to be derivatives of embryonic coelomic epithelium, we investigated serum CA-125 levels in patients with endometriosis. We observed that patients with stage II, III, and IV endometriosis (American Fertility Society classification [132]) had significantly elevated blood levels of CA-125 [125] (Fig. 2). This finding has been confirmed by other investigators [133,134]. The AFS score was significantly correlated with the degree of elevation in serum CA-125 [125]. Immunocytochemical studies demonstrated that endometriotic glands and stroma contain high membrane concentrations of CA-125.

Of particular interest is our recent observation that the change in CA-125 levels during and after treatment for endometriosis correlates well with other subjective and objective response parameters, such as pelvic pain and cul-de-sac nodularity. Figure 3 demonstrates the change in serum CA-125 levels in six patients with advanced endometriosis who were treated with total hysterectomy and bilateral oophorectomy. Figure 4 demonstrates the serum CA-125 concentrations and the AFS scores [132] in ten patients with endometriosis treated with danazol for 6 months who were laparoscoped before and after danazol treatment. The CA-125 assay is *not* a good screening test for

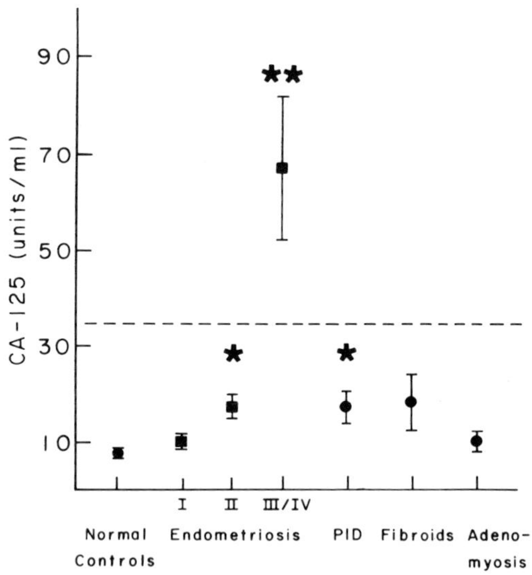

Fig. 2. Serum CA-125 concentrations in 146 patients undergoing diagnostic laparoscopy or laparotomy. Mean ± SEM. *p < 0.05, **p < 0.001 compared with controls. The normal controls were patients with visually normal pelvic organs at the time of diagnostic laparoscopy. Reproduced with the permission of the publisher, The American Fertility Society, Birmingham, AL [125].

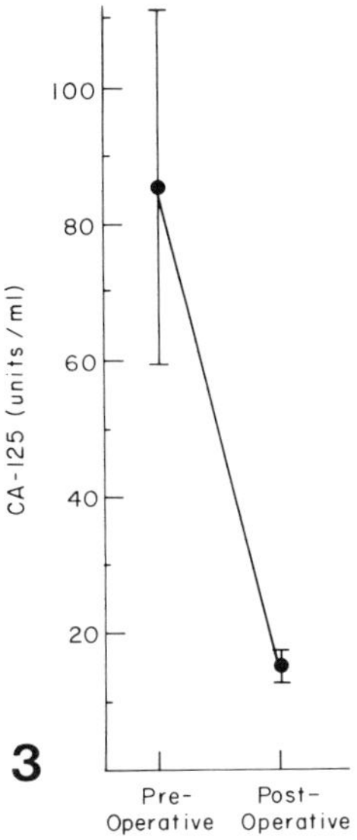

3

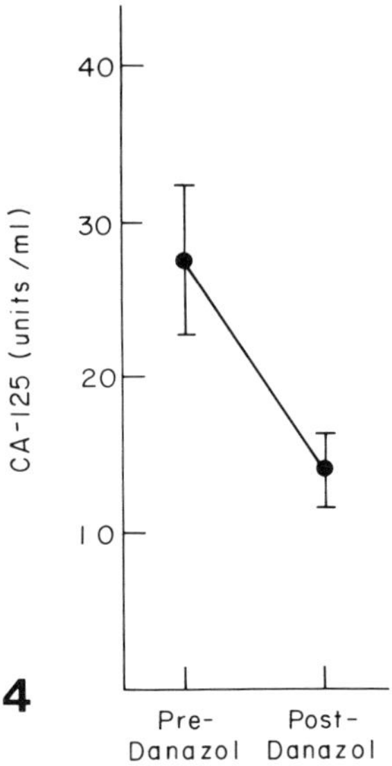

4

Fig. 3. Pre- and postoperative serum CA-125 concentrations in six patients with advanced endometriosis who had total abdominal hysterectomy-bilateral oophorectomy. Postoperative serum CA-125 concentration was measured 3 months after surgery. $^{+}p<0.02$.

Fig. 4. Serum CA-125 concentrations pre- and postdanazol therapy in ten patients with endometriosis. Patients were laparoscoped pre- and postdanazol therapy to monitor disease course. American Fertility Society endometriosis score pretherapy: 26, postherapy: 14.

endometriosis because of its *low* sensitivity. However, the measurement of serum CA-125 may prove to be a useful parameter of endometriosis disease activity. Clearly, a "blood test" for endometrioisis would represent a significant advance in gynecology.

REFERENCES

1. Karnaky KJ: The use of stilbestrol for endometriosis. South Med J 41:1109, 1948.
2. Kistner RW: The use of newer progestins in the treatment of endometriosis. Am J Obstet Gynecol 75:264, 1958.
3. Kistner RW: The treatment of endometriosis by inducing pseudopregnancy with ovarian hormones: a report of 58 cases. Fertil Steril 10:539, 1959.
4. Kistner RW: The use of steroidal substances in endometriosis. Clin Pharmacol Ther 1:525, 1960.
5. Dmowski WP, Cohen MR: Antigonadotropin (danazol) in the treatment of endometriosis. Am J Obstet Gynecol 130:41, 1978.

6. Barbieri RL, Evans S, Kistner RW: Danazol in the treatment of endometriosis: analysis of 100 cases with a 4-year follow-up. Fertil Steril 37:737, 1982.
7. Buttram VC, Reiter RC, Ward S: Treatment of endometriosis with danazol: report of a six year prospective study. Fertil Steril 43:353, 1985.
8. Meldrum DR: Clinical management of endometriosis with luteinizing hormone-releasing hormone analogues. Semin Reprod Endocrinol 3:371, 1985.
9. Janne O, Kauppila A, Kokko E: Estrogen and progestin receptors in endometriotic lesions: comparison with endometrial tissue. Am J Obstet Gynecol 141:562, 1981.
10. Tamaya T, Motoyama T, Ohono Y: Steroid receptor levels and histology of endometriosis and adenomysis. Fertil Steril 31:396, 1979.
11. Vihko R, Isotalo H, Kauppila A: Hormonal regulation of endometrium and endometriosis tissue. In Raynaud JP (ed): "Medical Management of Endometriosis." New York: Raven Press, p 79, 1984.
12. DiZerga GS, Barber DL, Hodgen GD: Endometriosis: role of ovarian steroids in initiation, maintenance and suppression. Fertil Steril 33:649, 1980.
13. Cunha GR: Stromal induction and specification of morphogenesis and cytodifferentiation of the epithelia of the Mullerian ducts and urogenital sinus during the development of the uterus and vagina in mice. J Exp Zool 196:361, 1976.
14. Cunha GR, Chung LWK, Shannon JM: Hormone induced morphogenesis and growth: role of mesenchymal-epithelial interactions. Recent Prog Horm Res 39:559, 1983.
15. Cunha GR, Bigsby RM, Cooke PS, Sugimura Y: Stromal-epithelial interactions in adult organs. Cell Differ 17:137, 1985.
16. Weed JC, Arguembourg PC: Endometriosis: can it produce an autoimmune response resulting in infertility? Clin Obstet Gynecol 23:3, 1980.
17. Haney AF, Muscato JJ, Weinberg JB: Peritoneal fluid cell populations in infertility patients. Fertil Steril 35:696, 1981.
18. Badaway SZ, Cuenca V, Marshall L, Munchibak R, Rivas AC, Coble DA: Cellular components in peritoneal fluid in infertile patients with and without endometriosis. Fertil Steril 42:704, 1984.
19. Kreiner D, Fromowitz FB, Richardson DA, Kenigsberg D: Endometrial immunofluorescence associated with endometriosis and pelvic inflammatory disease. Fertil Steril 464:243, 1986.
20. Kistner RW: Management of endometriosis in the infertile patient. Fertil Steril 26:1151, 1975.
21. Muse KN, Wilson EA: How does mild endometriosis cause infertility? Fertil Steril 38:145, 1982.
22. Seibel MM: Minimal pelvic endometriosis and infertility. Semin Reprod Endocrinol 3:307, 1985.
23. Seibel MM, Berger MJ, Weinstein FJK, Taymor ML: The effectiveness of danazol on subsequent fertility in minimal endometriosis. Fertil Steril 38:534, 1982.
24. Olive DL, Haney AF: Endometriosis-associated infertility: a critical review of therapeutic approaches. Obstet Gynecol Surv 41:538, 1986.
25. Davison C, Banks W, Fritz A: The absorption, distribution and metabolic fate of danazol in rats, monkeys and human volunteers. Arch Int Pharmacodyn Ther 221:294, 1976.
26. Rosi D, Neumann HC, Christiansen RG: Isolation, synthesis and biologic activity of five metabolites of danazol. J Med Chem 26:349, 1977.
27. Desaulles PA, Krahenbuhl C: Comparison of the anti-fertility and sex hormone activities of sex hormones and derivatives. Acta Endocrinol 47:444, 1964.

28. Barbieri RL, Lee H, Ryan KJ: Danazol binding to rat androgen, glucocorticoid, progesterone and estrogen receptors: correlation with biologic activity. Fertil Steril 31:181–186, 1979.
29. Chamness GC, Asch RN, Pauerstein CJ: Danazol binding and translocation of steroid receptors. Am J Obstet Gynecol 136:426–429, 1980.
30. Punnonen R, Lukola A: Competitive inhibition by danazol of progesterone and dihydrotestosterone binding to human uterine progestin and androgen receptors. Horm Metab Res 14:167–168, 1982.
31. Kokko E, Janne O, Kauppila A, Ronnberg L, Vihko R: Danazol has progestin-like actions on the human endometrium. Acta Endocrinol 99:588–593, 1982.
32. Tamaya T, Furuka N, Motoyama T, Boku S, Ohono Y, Okada N: Mechanism of antiprogestational action of synthetic steroids. Acta Endocrinol 88:190–198, 1978.
33. Jenkin G, Cookson CI, Thornburn GD: The interaction of human endometrial and myometrial steroid receptors with danazol. Clin Endocrinol 19:377–388, 1983.
34. Krey LC, Robbins R, McEwen BS: Danazol suppression of luteinizing hormone secretion: a role for danazol-androgen receptor interaction within the brain-pituitary complex. Fertil Steril 35:467–472, 1981.
35. Pugeat MM, Dunn JF, Rodbard D, Nisula BC: The significance of drug interactions with human TeBG and CBG under physiological conditions: a new approach. J Steroid Biochem 15:487–490, 1981.
36. Pugeat MM, Dunn JF, Nisula BC: Transport of steroid hormones: interaction of 70 drugs with testosterone-binding globulin and corticosteroid-binding globulin in human plasma. J Clin Endocrinol Metab 53:69–75, 1981.
37. Dmowski WP, Scholer HFL, Mahesh VB, Greenblatt RB: Danazol, a synthetic steroid derivative with interesting physiologic properties. Fertil Steril 22:9–18, 1971.
38. Wentz AC, Jones GS, Sapp KC, King TM: Progestational activity of danazol in the human female subject. Am J Obstet Gynecol 126:378–384, 1976.
39. Kokko E: Progestin-like effects of danazol on rabbit uterus. Endocrinology 112:1110, 1983.
40. Summary of basis for FDA approval of danazol. NDA 17557, Food and Drug Administration, USPHS, DHEW, 1975.
41. Allen JK, Fraser IS: Cholesterol, high-density lipoproteins and danazol. J Clin Endocrinol Metab 53:149, 1981.
42. Luciano AA, Hauser KC, Chapler FK, Sherman BM: Effects of danazol on plasma lipid and lipoprotein levels in healthy women with endometriosis. Am J Obstet Gynecol 145:422, 1983.
43. Fahraeus L, Larsson-Cohn V, Ljingberg S, Wallentin L: Profound alterations of lipoprotein metabolism during danazol treatment in premenopausal women. Fertil Steril 42:52, 1984.
44. Wynn V: Metabolic effects of danazol. J Int Med Res 5:25, 1977,
45. Laurell CB, Rannevik G: A comparison of plasma protein changes induced by danazol, pregnancy and estrogens. J Clin Endocrinol Metab 49:719–725, 1979.
46. Ahn YS, Harrington WJ, Simon SR: Danazol for the treatment of idiopathic thrombocytopenic purpura. N Engl J Med 308:1396, 1983.
47. Agnello V, Pariser K, Gell J: Preliminary observations on danazol therapy of systemic lupus erythematosus: effects on DNA antibodies, thrombocytopenia, and complement. J Rheumatol 10:682, 1983.

48. Nilsson B, Sodergard R, Damber MG, vonSchoultz B: Danazol and gestagen displacement of testosterone and influence of sex-hormone binding globulin capacity. Fertil Steril 38:48–53, 1982.
49. Schwarz S, Hintner H, Tappeiner G: Endocrinologic study in 4 patients with hereditary angioneurotic edema before and during danazol therapy: effects of sex-hormone binding globulin. Acta Endocrinol S225:114A, 1979.
50. Nilsson B, Sodergard R, Damber MG, Damber JE, Vonschouler B: Free testosterone levels during danazol therapy. Fertil Steril 39:505–509, 1983.
51. Barbieri RL, Canick JA, Makris A, Davies IJ, Rayan KJ: Danazol inhibits steroidogenesis. Fertil Steril 28:809, 1977.
52. Barbieri RL, Canick JA, Ryan KJ: Danazol inhibits steroidogenesis in the rat testis in vitro. Endocrinology 101:1676–1681, 1977.
53. Barbieri RL, Osathanondh R, Canick JA, Stillman RJ, Ryan KJ: Danazol inhibits human adrenal 21-and 11 β-hydroxylation in vitro. Steroids 35:251–263, 1980.
54. Asch RH, Fernandez EO, Siler-Khodr TM, Bartke A, Pauerstein CJ: Mechanism of induction of luteal phase defects by danazol. Am J Obstet Gynecol 136:932–940, 1980.
55. Wentz AC, Sapp KC: Danazol as a luteolytic agent. Fertil Steril 19:23–25, 1978.
56. Steingold KA, Lu JKH, Judd HL, Meldrum DR: Danazol inhibits steroidogenesis by the human ovary in vivo. Fertil Steril 45:649, 1986.
57. Stillman RJ, Fencl M, Schiff I, Barbieri RL, Tulchinsky D: Inhibition of adrenal steroidogenesis by danazol in vivo. Fertil Steril 33:401–406, 1980.
58. Castro-Magana M, Cherovanky T, Collipp PJ, Ghavami-Maibodi Z, Angulo M, Stewart C: Transient adrenogenital syndrome due to exposure to danazol in utero. Am J Dis Child 135:1032–1034, 1981.
59. Reyniak JV, Gurpide E: Effect of danazol on gonadal steroidogenesis in patients with a complete form of testicular feminization. Am J Obstet Gynecol 142:479–481, 1982.
60. Duck SC, Katayama KP: Danazol may cause female pseudohermaphroditism. Fertil Steril 35:230, 1981.
61. Shaw RW, Farquhar JW: Female pseudohermaphroditism associated with danazol exposure in utero. Case report. Br J Obstet Gynaecol 91:386, 1984.
62. Peress MR, Kreutner AK, Mathur RS, Williamson HO: Female pseudohermaphroditism with somatic chromosomal anomaly in association with in utero exposure to danazol. Am J Obstet Gynecol 142:708, 1982.
63. Kingsbury AC: Danazol and fetal masculinization: a warning. Med J Aust 153:410, 1985.
64. Quagliarello J, Greco MA: Danazol and urogenital sinus formation in pregnancy. Fertil Steril 43:939, 1985.
65. Ward GD: Dosage aspects of danazol therapy in the treatment of endometriosis. Postgrad Med J 55(Suppl 5):75–78, 1979.
66. Biberoglu KO, Behrman SJ: Dosage aspects of danazol therapy in endometriosis: short-term and long-term effectiveness. Am J Obstet Gynecol 139:645–654, 1981.
67. Dickey RP, Taylor SN, Curole DN: Serum estradiol and danazol. I. Endometriosis response, side effects, administration interval, concurrent spironolactone and dexamethasone. Fertil Steril 42:709–716, 1984.
68. Mercaitis PA, Peaper RE, Schwartz PA: Effect of danazol on vocal pitch: a case study. Obstet Gynecol 65:131–135, 1985.
69. Wardle PG, Whitehead MI, Mills RP: Nonreversible and wide ranging vocal changes after treatment with danazol. Br Med J 287:946–948, 1983.

70. Graham RL, Gambrell RD: Changes in thyroid function tests during danazol therapy, Obstet Gynecol 55:395–397, 1980.
71. Barbieri RL: Danazol and thyroid function. Ann Intern Med 92:133, 1980.
72. Bretza JA, Novey HS, Vaziri ND, Warner AS: Hypertension: a complication of danazol therapy. Arch Intern Med 140:1379–1380, 1980.
73. Duff P, Mayer AR: Generalized alopecia: an unusual complication of danazol therapy. Am J Obstet Gynecol 141:349–350, 1980.
74. Goulbourne IA, MacLeod DAD: An interaction between danazol and warfarin. Br J Obstet Gynaecol 88:950–951, 1981.
75. Pearson K, Zimmerman HJ: Danazol and liver damage. Lancet 1:645–646, 1980.
76. Ronnberg L, Ylostalo P: Treatment of pulmonary endometriosis with danazol. Acta Obstet Gynecol Scand 60:77, 1981.
77. Gardner B, Whitaker RH: The use of danazol for ureteral obstruction caused by endometriosis. J Urol 125:117–118, 1981.
78. Pittaway DE, Daniell JF, Maxson WS, Winifield AC, Wentz AC: Recurrence of ureteral obstruction caused by endometriosis after danazol therapy. Am J Obstet Gynecol 143:720–722, 1982.
79. Friedlander RL: The treatment of endometriosis with danazol. J Reprod Med 10:197–199, 1973.
80. Grennblatt RB, Tzingonnis V: Danazol treatment of endometriosis: long-term follow-up. Fertil Steril 32:518–520, 1979.
81. Dmowski WP, Cohen MR: Treatment of endometriosis with an antigonadotropin danazol. Obstet Gynecol 46:147–154, 1975.
82. Puelo JG, Hammond CB: Conservative treatment of endometriosis externa: the effects of danazol therapy. Fertil Steril 40:164, 1983.
83. Lauersen NH, Wilson KH, Birnbaum S: Danazol: an antigonadotropic agent in the treatment of pelvic endometriosis. Am J Obstet Gynecol 123:742–747, 1975.
84. Barbieri RL, Ryan KJ: Danazol: endocrine pharmacology and therapeutic applications. Am J Obstet Gynecol 141:453–463, 1981.
85. Deltour G, Azadian-Boulanger G, Nelson J, Sakiz E: Tolerance and contraceptive efficacy of gestrinone in 800 patients in the United States from 1975 to 1978. In Raynaud JP (ed): "Medical Management of Endometriosis." New York: Raven Press, pp 223–231, 1984.
86. Sakiz G, Azadian-Boulanger G, Lavaque F, Raynaud JP: A new approach to estrogen-free contraception based on progesterone receptor blockage by mid-cycle administration of ethyl norgestrinone (R2323). Contraception 10:467–474, 1974.
87. Mora G, Faudes A, Pastore U: Clinical evaluation of an oral progestin contraceptive, R-2323, 5 mg., administered at weekly intervals. Contraception 10:145–157, 1974.
88. Coutinho E: Clinical experience with implant contraception. Contraception 18:411–427, 1978.
89. Azadian-Boulanger G, Secchi J, Tournemine C, Sakiz E, Vige P, Henrian R: Hormonal activity profiles of drugs for endometriosis therapy. In Raynaud JP (ed): "Medical Management of Endometriosis." New York: Raven Press, pp 125–148, 1984.
90. Moguilewsky M, Philibert D: Dynamics of receptor interactions of danazol and gestrinone in the rat: correlations with biological activities. In Raynaud JP (ed): "Medical Management of Endometriosis." New York: Raven Press, pp 163–181, 1984.
91. Chalbos D, Bardon S, Vignon F, Rocheford H: Use of hormone-responsive cell lines to study the mechanism of action of progestins and antiprogestins. In Raynaud JP (ed): "Medical Management of Endometriosis." New York: Raven Press, pp 53–65, 1984.

92. Pugeat M, Nicholas B, Tourniaire J, Forest MG: Interaction of gestrinone with human plasma steriod-binding proteins. In Raynaud JP (ed): "Medical Management of Endometriosis." New York: Raven Press, pp 183–192, 1984.
93. Belghmi K, Michel F, Nicholas JC, Descomps B, de Paulet AC: Inhibition of enzymes involved in steroid and prostanoid metabolism by steroids used in endometriosis therapy. In Raynaud JP (ed): "Medical Management of Endometriosis." New York: Raven Press, pp 9–96, 1984.
94. Proulx L, Labrie F, Veilleux R, Azadian-Boulanger G: Actions of progestins and androgens at the hypothalamo-adenohypophyseal level in the female rat. In Raynaud JP (ed): "Medical Management of Endometriosis." New York: Raven Press, pp 149–161, 1984.
95. Mettler L, Semm K: Three-step therapy of genital endometriosis in cases of human infertility with lynestrenol, danazol or gestrinone administration in the second step. In Raynaud JP (ed): "Medical Management of Endometriosis." New York: Raven Press, pp 233–247, 1984.
96. Coutinho EM: Treatment of endometriosis with gestrinone (R2323), a synthetic antiestrogen, antiprogesterone. Am J Obstet Gynecol 144:895, 1982.
97. Treadway DR, Mishell DR: Effect of a once weekly oral contraceptive upon gonadotropin and gonadal steroid levels. Contraception 10:159–169, 1974.
98. Victor A, Johansson EDB: The effect of weekly administration of an oral progestogen - R-2323 - on the ovarian function. Contraception 12:89–94, 1975.
99. Spellacy WN, Buhi WC, Dumdaugh VA, Birk SA: The effects of a once-a-week steroid contraceptive (R2323) on lipid and carbohydrate metabolism in women during three months of use. Fertil Steril 30:289–292, 1978.
100. Spellacy WN, Mahan CS, Buhi MS, Dumbaugh RN, Birk SA: Blood glucose, insulin, cholesterol and triglyceride levels in women treated for six months with the weekly oral contraceptive R2323. Contraception 18:121–126, 1978.
101. Vickery BM: Comparison of the potential for therapeutic utilities with gonadotropin-releasing hormone agonists and antagonists. Endocr Rev 7:115–124, 1986.
102. Meldrum DR, Chang RJ, Lu W, Rivier J, Judd HL: Medical oophorectomy using a long-acting GnRH agonist: a possible new approach to the treatment of endometriosis. J Clin Endocrinol Metab 54:1081–1083, 1982.
103. The Leuprolide Study Group: Leuprolide versus diethylstilbestrol for metastatic prostate cancer. N Engl J Med 311:1281, 1984.
104. Nestor JJ: Development of agonistic LHRH analogs. In Vickery BH, Nestor JJ, Hafez ESE (eds): "LHRH and Its Analogs: Contraceptive and Therapeutic Applications." Lancaster, England: MTP Press, pp 3–10, 1984.
105. Werlin LB, Hodgen GD: Gonadotropin-releasing hormone agonist suppresses ovulation, menses and endometriosis in monkeys: an individualized intermittent regimen. J Clin Endocrinol Metab 56:844–846, 1983.
106. Jones RC: The effect of a luteinizing hormone releasing hormone (LRH) agonist (Wy-40,972) levonorgestrel, danazol and ovariectomy on experimental endometriosis in the rat. Acta Endorinol 106:282–288, 1984.
107. Meldrum DR, Tsao Z, Monroe SE, Braustein GD, Sladek J, Lu JKH, Vale W, Rivier J, Judd HL, Chang RL: Stimulation of LH fragments with reduced bioactivity following GnRH agonist administration in women. J Clin Endocrinol Metabl 58:755–757, 1984.
108. Jennes L, Stumpf WE, Con PE: Intracellular pathways of electron-dense GnRH analogs in cultured pituitary gonadotropins. In Programs and Abstracts, 65th Annual Meeting of the Endocrine Society, San Antonio, June 8–10, 1983, p 155.

109. Lemay A, Quesnel G: Potential new treatment of endometriosis: reversible inhibition of pituitary-ovarian function by chronic intranasal administration of a luteinizing hormone-releasing hormone (LH-RH) agonist. Fertil Steril 38:376–379, 1982.
110. Lemay A, Maheux R, Fauve N, Jean C, Fazekas AT: Reversible hypogonadism induced by a luteinizing hormone-releasing hormone (LH-RH) agonist (Buserelin) as a new therapeutic approach for endometriosis. Fertil Steril 41:863–871, 1984.
111. Pring DW, Maresh M, Fraser AC: Luteinising hormone releasing hormone agonist in women with endometriosis. Br Med J 287:1718–1719, 1983.
112. Shaw RW, Fraser HM, Boyle H: Intranasal treatment with luteinising hormone releasing hormone agonist in women with endometriosis. Br Med J 287:1667–1669, 1983.
113. Schriock E, Monroe SE, Henzl M, Jaffe R: Treatment of endometriosis with a potent agonist of gonadotropin-releasing hormone (Nafarelin). Fertil Steril 44:583–588, 1985.
114. DeFazio J, Meldrum DR, Lu JKH, Vale WW, Rivier JE, Judd HL, Chang RL: Acute ovarian responses to a long-acting agonist of GnRH in ovulatory women and women with polycystic ovarian disease. Fertil Steril 44:453–459, 1985.
115. Frazer HM, Sandow J: Suppression of follicular maturation by infusion of a luteinizing hormone-releasing hormone agonist starting during the late luteal phase in the stump-tailed macaque monkey. J Clin Endocinol Metab 60:579–584, 1985.
116. Schiff I, Tulchinsky D, Cramer D, Ryan K: Medroxyprogesterone in the treatment of postmenopausal symptoms. JAMA 244:1443–1445, 1980.
117. Andreyko J, Blumenfeld Z, Marshall L, Hrieak H, Conn L, Monroe S: Treatment of uterine leiomyomata with a GnRH agonist. Society for Gynecologic Investigation, 1986, p 96.
118. Meldrum DR: Management of endometriosis with gonadotropin-releasing hormone agonists. Fertil Steril 44:581–582, 1985.
119. Noble AD, Letchworth AT: Medical treatment of endometriosis: a comparative trial. Postgrad Med J 55(Suppl 5):37–40, 1979.
120. Hammond MG, Hammond CB, Parker RT: Conservative treatment of endometriosis externa: the effects of methyltestosterone therapy. Fertil Steril 29:651–654, 1978.
121. Katayama KP, Manuel M, Jones HW, Jones GS: Methyltestosterone treatment of infertility associated with pelvic endometriosis. Fertil Steril 27:83–86, 1976.
122. Preston SN, Campbell HB: Pelvic endometriosis, treatment with methyltestosterone. Obstet Gynecol 2:152–157, 1953.
123. Mettler L, Sem K: Three-step therapy of genital endometriosis in cases of human infertility with lynestrenol, danazol or gestrinone administration in the second step. In Raynaud JP (ed): "Medical Management of Endometriosis." New York: Raven Press, pp 233–247, 1984.
124. Moghissi KS, Boyce CR: Management of endometriosis with oral medroxyprogesterone acetate. Obstet Gynecol 47:265–267, 1976.
125. Barbieri RL, Niloff JM, Bast RC, Schaetzl E, Kistner RW, Knapp RC: Elevated serum concentrations of CA-125 in patients with advanced endometriosis. Fertil Steril 45:630, 1986.
126. Barbieri RL: CA-125 in patients with endometriosis. Fertil Steril 45:767, 1986.
127. Bast RC Jr, Freeney M, Lazarus H, Nadler LM, Colvin RB, Knapp RC; Reactivity of a monoclonal antibody with human ovarian carcinoma. J Clin Invest 68:1331, 1981.
128. Kabawat SE, Bast RC Jr, Welch WR, Knapp RC, Colvin RB: Immunopathologic characterization of a monoclonal antibody that recognizes common surface antigens in human ovarian tumors of serous, endometrioid and clear cell type. Am J Clin Pathol 79:98, 1983.

129. Kabawat SE, Bast RC Jr, Bhan AK, Welch WR, Knapp RC, Colvin RB: Tissue distribution of a coelomic-epithelium-related antigen recognized by the monoclonal antibody OC-125. Int J Gynecol Pathol 2:275, 1983.
130. Masuho Y, Zalutsky M, Knapp RC, Bast RC Jr: Interaction of monoclonal antibodies with cell surface antigens of human ovarian carcinoma. Cancer Res 44:2813, 1984.
131. Bast RC Jr, Klug TL, St. John E, Jenison E, Niloff JM, Lazarus H, Berkowitz RS, Leavitt T, Griffiths CT, Parker L, Zurawski VR Jr, Knapp RC: A radioimunoassay using a monoclonal antibody to monitor the course of epithelial ovarian cancer. N Engl J Med 309:883, 1983.
132. The American Fertility Society: Classification of endometriosis. Fertil Steril 32:633, 1979.
133. Giudice LC, Jacobs A, Pineda J, Bell CE, Lippmann L: Serum levels of CA-125 in patients with endometriosis. Fertil Steril 45:876, 1986.
134. Patton PE, Field CS, Harms RW, Coulam CB: CA-125 levels in endometriosis. Fertil Steril 45:770, 1986.

Endometriosis, pages 141–160

Chapter 8
Conservative Surgery for Endometriosis

L. Russell Malinak, M.D., and James M. Wheeler, M.D.

Department of Obstetrics and Gynecology, Baylor College of Medicine, Houston, Texas 77030 (L.R.M.); Department of Obstetrics and Gynecology, Yale University, New Haven, Connecticut (J.M.W.)

INTRODUCTION

Despite advances in the development of effective medical therapy and popularization of in vitro fertilization, "the surgical treatment of endometriosis remains the 'gold standard' for the therapy of this disease. . . . There is certainly not yet reason to believe that surgery should be replaced as primary therapy for endometriosis under suitable circumstances" [1]. This discussion of the surgical treatment of endometriosis will emphasize the: 1) Individualization of therapy and proper case selection for conservative surgery, 2) Indications, technique, and results of conservative surgery via laparoscopy and laparotomy, 3) Use of adjuvant operations (e.g., presacral neurectomy) and medications (e.g., danazol), and 4) Results of treatment in regard to pregnancy and reoperation rates.

The literature and original research presented in this chapter are current as of September, 1986, and must be collated with most recent information available. Referencing for each section is meant to represent a consensus of current opinion; our own personal opinions and recommendations are presented as such if they differ from collective thought. Major areas of discussion include mention of a selected review article for more indepth study.

INDIVIDUALIZATION OF THERAPY

The Surgical Staging of Endometriosis

To properly decide upon the most appropriate form of treatment for the individual patient, the clinician must depend on treatment choices proven efficacious tempered by his/her own personal experience. Prior to the institution of any treatment of endometriosis, the disease must first be definitively diagnosed and surgically staged by laparoscopy. Proper staging necessitates use of a classification system—an area of clinical research that is rapidly evolving [2]. At this writing, the recommended morphologic classification of endometriosis is the "Revised American Fertility Society Classification" (Chapter 5)[3]. This classification represents the collective opinion of several respected clinicians experienced in the treatment of women with endometriosis; our input into the process included a recommendation to weigh adnexal adhesions heavily in deference to the total "mass" of endometriosis. It is hoped that the classification will permit "more interpretable data collection, more objective evaluation of therapeutics, and more justifiable prognostication for patients with endometriosis" [4]. The greatest contribution of this classification is the concept of a permanent detailed record of each woman's pelvis; reprints of the classification form are readily available from the AFS. Ultimately, empirically derived classification systems will be adjusted to reflect knowledge gained from analysis of the relationship of individual anatomic areas to prognosis for pregnancy and recurrence [5]. Until a proposed classification is demonstrably and reproducibly capable of predicting pregnancy and recurrence rates, the operative findings of each patient should be detailed on one of the AFS forms rather than simply recorded in the charts as "Stage X" disease.

Overview of Treatment Options—Use of the Treatment Algorithm

Individualization of therapy is based largely upon the stage of disease, the somatic complaints, and the reproductive goals of each woman. For purpose of triage to treatment, patients may be divided into three general categories: 1) Women with endometriosis-associated infertility, with or without somatic symptoms, 2) Women with pelvic pain who desire preservation of their fertility potential, and 3) Women with somatic complaints who have completed their childbearing. Based on these three patient groups and the four stages of endometriosis encompassing the revised AFS classification system, a clinically useful algorithm is presented in Figure 1.

The initial treatment of choice for most infertile women with Stage I (minimal) or Stage II (mild) endometriosis is expectant management (cf. Seibel 1985 for review) [6]. This review fails to demonstrate a marked advantage of medical or surgical therapy over expectant management of infertile women with mild endometriosis.

It is important to note that expectant treatment is not synonymous with "no treatment." Complete infertility investigation is warranted, and correction of concomitant factors is indicated (e.g., anovulation, male factor). The couple is followed closely; medical or surgical treatment is indicated if pregnancy does not occur with 6 to 12 months of expectant therapy, or if the couple prefers immediate, more active treatment.

ENDOMETRIOSIS TREATMENT ALGORITHM

	Desires Childbearing		Childbearing Complete
CHIEF COMPLAINT	INFERTILITY	PELVIC PAIN	PELVIC PAIN
STAGES I & II	1. EXPECTANT Tx 2. LAPAROSCOPIC T x 2. MEDICAL T x 3. CSEL ± PSN 3. IVF/ET	1. LAPAROSCOPIC Tx 2. MEDICAL Tx 3. CSEL + PSN	1. LAPAROSCOPIC Tx 2. MEDICAL Tx 3. TAH ± BSO 3. CSEL + PSN
STAGE III	1. LAPAROSCOPIC T x 1. CSEL ± PSN 2. MEDICAL T x 3. IVF/ET	1. LAPAROSCOPIC Tx 2. CSEL + PSN 3. MEDICAL Tx	1. LAPAROSCOPIC Tx 2. MEDICAL Tx 3. TAH ± BSO 3. CSEL + PSN
STAGE IV	1. CSEL + PERIOPERATIVE MEDICAL Tx 2. CSEL ALONE 3. LAPAROSCOPIC Tx + POSTOPERATIVE MEDICAL Tx 4. IVF/ET	1. CSEL + PSN + PERIOPERATIVE MEDICAL Tx 2. MEDICAL Tx 3. LAPAROSCOPIC Tx + MEDICAL Tx	1. TAH ± BSO 1. CSEL + PSN + MEDICAL T x 2. LAPAROSCOPIC Tx + MEDICAL Tx

CSEL — conservative surgery for endometriosis at laparotomy
PSN — presacral neurectomy
TAH — total abdominal hysterectomy
BSO — bilateral salpingo-oophorectomy
IVF/ET - in vitro fertilization/embryo transfer
"±" — indicates adjunctive treatment option based on individual patient findings

Fig. 1. Treatment options for patients with endometriosis. First, determine the patient's interest in childbearing and her major complaint. The therapeutic options are listed for each AFS classification by order of preference; two treatments at the same rank have similar levels of preference.

The next line of treatment involves a choice between medical therapy and laparoscopic surgical therapy. Women with somatic complaints should not be treated expectantly, regardless of their desire for fertility; their first line of treatment involves the same choice between medical and laparoscopic therapy. Medical therapy is covered in detail in Chapter 7. At this writing, danazol is the most available and widely used form of medical therapy [7]. However, analogs of gonadotropin-releasing hormone (GnRH) show outstanding promise [8,9]. For women not currently seeking conception, some authors recommend suppression with a low-dose estrogen-progestin oral contraceptive [10]. However, more recent epidemiologic data from a collaborative study show a higher than expected rate of oral contraceptive use in women with endometriosis [11].

Laparoscopic therapy may be performed immediately at diagnosis in Stages I, II, and III endometriosis in women with infertility or somatic complaints. If therapeutic laparoscopic equipment is not available, or if preoperative counseling of the patient reveals her preference for expectant or medical therapy, laparoscopic treatment may be deferred. Whereas it is well established that the first conservative laparotomy for endometriosis offers the best chances of success [12,13], the effects of repeated laparoscopic surgery are unknown. Nevertheless, many experts feel that the equipment necessary for laparoscopic therapy should be available at every diagnostic laparoscopy for infertility or pelvic pain.

Conservative surgery for endometriosis at laparotomy (CSEL) is indicated in Stages I and II disease only if medical or laparoscopic surgery fails to relieve pelvic pain or if endometriosis recurs in a persistently infertile patient. CSEL remains the treatment of choice for Stage IV endometriosis, and is an appropriate treatment option in Stage III disease. More specific indications, technique, and use of component procedures such as presacral neurectomy are discussed in the following section devoted to CSEL.

No discussion of the treatment of endometriosis today is complete without a discussion of the role of in vitro fertilization (IVF). Dr. Howard Jones has stated that "the time may be at hand to consider the possibility of proceeding with IVF as definitive treatment when a patient with mild or moderate endometriosis is over 35 years of age, regardless of prior therapy" [1]. In the Norfolk experience with 62 patients (85 cycles) between September, 1980, and December, 1984, an excellent per cycle pregnancy rate of 48.7% was reported in patients with minimal and mild endometriosis [14]. Unfortunately, women with moderate and severe endometriosis had only a 15.9% per cycle pregnancy rate [14], which is quite a bit lower than the overall success rate of 31% [1]. In vitro fertilization offers another successful treatment modality for the infertile woman with endometriosis. Due to the possible stimulation of endometriosis on hyperstimulation protocols, the lack of benefit for the common accompaniment of pelvic pain, the expense, and overall limited success, in vitro fertilization should be considered in most cases only after more traditional therapy has been exhausted.

Hysterectomy is becoming less of a necessity, owing to the successes of medical and conservative surgical approaches. It remains the most definitive chance for "cure," and is indicated in those women with any stage of disease in whom more conservative therapy has failed, or in those women who have completed childbearing and do not wish to preserve their uterus.

Having reviewed our approach to treatment decisions in this disease, the proper context is established for the discussion of the surgical treatment of endometriosis.

SURGICAL TECHNIQUES AND RESULTS

Laparoscopic Treatment

Laparoscopy has become one of the most commonly performed operations in gynecology, particularly in the evaluation and treatment of the infertile woman (cf. Corson 1979 [15] for review).

Initially a diagnostic tool, therapeutic laparoscopic maneuvers have quickly become a well-accepted mode of treatment of endometriosis and pelvic adhesions. In fact, DeCherney has predicted the "obituary of laparotomy for pelvic reconstructive surgery," having been supplanted by laparoscopic surgery [16].

As mentioned above, laparoscopy is the method of choice in diagnosing and staging endometriosis. Because of the more frequent use of laparoscopy in the evaluation of infertility and pelvic pain, surgeons are diagnosing more cases of endometriosis in earlier stages. Furthermore, the more frequent operative evaluation of the pelvis may reveal unsuspected endometriosis; a recent study of patients undergoing reversal of bilateral tubal sterilization revealed an 18.4% prevalence of endometriosis [18]. Laparoscopic biopsies will become even more important in the diagnosis and posttreatment follow-up of women with endometriosis.

Before the gynecologist makes the transition from laparoscopic diagnostician to surgical therapist, it is absolutely imperative that he become comfortable with the use of two- and three-puncture techniques [19,20]. The laparoscopic surgeon must be primarily responsible for the operating laparoscope and its accessories; he should know the technical aspects of the equipment better than anyone in the operating theater. He must be well versed in all modalities available for the operating laparoscope—even though he may choose to vaporize endometriosis with the carbon dioxide laser, use of the bipolar or unipolar cautery may be necessary to control unexpected bleeding. Each surgeon must acquire appropriate skills prior to "pushing the limits of what he can accomplish laparoscopically" [19], as in the laparoscopic treatment of 7 cm ovarian endometriomas or bladder implants [21]. The location and schedule of recommended courses in laparoscopic surgery and laser techniques may be obtained from the American Fertility Society and the American College of Obstetricians and Gynecologists. Following completion of such courses, it is recommended that the learning laparoscopist arrange an apprenticeship with an experienced endoscopic surgeon.

Since manipulation of the ovaries is routine in operative laparoscopy, the patient should be scheduled during the proliferative phase of her cycle to avoid the risk of bleeding associated with corpora lutea. Informed consent for the operation must include the risk of laparotomy to complete the procedure or to treat complications. Furthermore, the patient should have appropriate preoperative orders and anesthetic consultation as if she would require laparotomy.

At laparoscopy, there are several modes of destruction of endometriosis or adhesions listed in historical order: 1) Blunt dissection via second puncture probe, 2) Electrical cautery—unipolar and bipolar, 3) Carbon dioxide (CO_2) laser, and 4) Investigational lasers including the argon and the neodymium: yttrium, aluminum, garnet (Nd:YAG) lasers.

The only current use of the first method—blunt dissection—is in early second-look laparoscopy following laparotomy for tubal disease [22,23] or endometriosis [24]. Although critics might say that sharp dissection is preferable, blunt dissection is often inadvertent, owing to the very filmy nature of adhesions 12–16 days after laparotomy [24].

The Europeans Frangenheim [25] and Semm [26] were among the first proponents of electrocauterization of endometriosis via the laparoscope in the early 1970s. Eward [27] was the first of several American authors [27–30] describing cauterization of endometriosis at laparoscopy, sometimes in association with danazol therapy [30]. Daniell [30] reported a 67% conception rate in 66 patients with mild and moderate endometriosis treated with unipolar electrocautery, 90% of whom conceived within 6 months of laparoscopic treatment. An improvement in pain was reported by his patients as well [30].

The technique of cautery is perhaps the most established therapeutic modality in laparoscopy because of its early and continued use in tubal sterilization. Although bipolar cautery is without question safer when burning tubes, the unipolar cautery continues to have many uses in the treatment of endometriosis and adhesions. Flat or slightly raised areas of endometriosis are more amenable to a unipolar type of surface burn. Should dissection of adhesions produce brisk bleeding, this can best be handled by expeditious application of unipolar cautery. Following cauterization of vessels, microscissors can be used to divide coagulated adhesions safely. Cautery—in particular unipolar—should be avoided in areas near bowel, bladder, ureter, and broad ligaments as control of depth of tissue destruction is much less than that with the carbon dioxide laser.

Laser in Infertility Surgery

Following the first description of the use of the carbon dioxide laser intraabdominally for female reconstructive pelvic surgery in 1974 [31], laser therapy seemed to offer important technical advantages in comparative studies with electrocautery [32]. Of the many lasers studied in various surgical fields, three have been applied to gynecology—the carbon dioxide, the argon, and the neodymium:yttrium-aluminum-garnet (Nd:YAG). As an energy form, each laser has a specific wave length, producing different physical characteristics and tissue effects that are integral to its clinical applicability (Table I; cf. Daniell [33] for review). The carbon dioxide laser allows vaporization and precise incision of tissues with a very shallow depth of tissue destruction. Thus, the carbon dioxide laser has been the dominant laser form used in infertility surgery.

The biophysics of the carbon dioxide laser is a subject suitable for a separate chapter; interested readers are encouraged to read more in available reviews [33,34]. There are certain properties of the carbon dioxide laser, however, that are pertinent to the gynecologic surgeon and will be presented here [33]: 1) The energy is highly absorbed by nonreflective solids and liquids, most notably water. In water, the radiant energy is absorbed almost completely at a depth of 100 μm from the surface; 2) The beam is absorbed by tissues of all colors; 3) Radiant energy is converted efficiently to heat; tissue is vaporized by instantaneous boiling of cellular water. The energy is not known to cause residual genetic mutation of the cells; 4) There is minimal scattering of the beam at point of impact; some cellular damage from steam expansion occurs up to 500 μm from the laser impact; 5) The laser beam is efficiently reflected by mirrors or highly polished metals; 6) The energy of the beam may be focused to a spot diameter of less than 1 mm with minimal energy loss; it is this focusing that allows calculation of the clinically useful, "power density"; 7) Carbon dioxide laser systems are relatively compact and can operate from an ordinary electrical outlet; and 8) As carbon dioxide lasers vaporize rather coagulate, it is difficult to stop bleeding from vessels. Occluded vessels up to 2.0 mm can be sealed, compared to the 0.5 mm vessels that can be sealed if blood flow continues.

TABLE I. Comparison of Currently Used Lasers in Infertility Surgery

Characteristics	CO_2	Argon	Nd:YAG
Wave length	10.6 mm	0.5 mm	1.06 mm
Tissue effect	Vaporization	Coagulation	Coagulation
Depth of tissue effect	0.1 mm	0.5 mm	4 mm
Tissue effect dependent on color	No	Yes	Yes
Absorbance by water	Strong	None	Slight
Beam scatter	None	Slight	Moderate
Requires fiber	No	Yes	Yes

The most clinically useful application of the biophysics of the carbon dioxide laser is the adjustment of power density depending on specific surgical tasks. Power density changes with the spot size and the radiant energy of the beam; the smaller the spot size (i.e., the more focused the beam) and the higher the emitted energy, the greater the power density. The greater the power density, the more the laser behaves as a surgical knife in its ability to cleave tissues. With larger spot sizes ("defocusing" the beam) and lower energy settings, more hemostasis and tissue coagulation will occur. A typical setting for hemostasis is a 1 cm spot size and an output of 5 watts for a power density of 500 watts/cm2. Power densities up to 12,000 watts/cm2 are used for incisional purposes.

Carbon dioxide lasers have been used intraabdominally for over a decade on thousands of patients [33]. There was been a very good safety record, with the reported documented injuries being $< 0.5\%$. Examples of accidents that can occur include a malaligned aiming Helium:Neon (He:Ne) beam, inadvertent reflection off an instrument, ignition of flammable drapes or sponges, and burning the fingers of the assistant. The Nd:YAG and argon lasers present more serious safety hazards because of their greater beam backscatter. Surgeons and hospitals must insure that all precautions possible are taken to protect the patient and the operative team from laser injury.

The first use of the carbon dioxide laser laparoscope was reported by Bruhat et al., in 1979 [35]. Numerous reports have claimed safe and effective treatment for endometriosis using carbon dioxide laser laparoscopy [19–21,36–39]. In a literature review of 113 patients treated as of 1985, Daniell [20] noted an overall pregnancy rate of 38%. In his own series of 58 patients, he reported a 50% conception rate and 72% incidence of pain relief [20]. The most recent report on carbon dioxide laser laparoscopy [21] relates the following term pregnancy rates per AFS stage of disease: Stage I—75% (18/24 patients); Stage II—63% (32/51); Stage III—42% (8/19); Stage IV—50% (4/8). As described above, Nezhat's [21] preliminary report contains too few cases to draw conclusions particularly regarding efficacy and safety in Stage III and IV disease. Perhaps the greatest contribution of this report is the description of a videomonitoring technique similar to the method used for arthroscopy [21]; this so-called videolaseroscopy avoids the often limiting back strain of a prolonged laparoscopic procedure and allows permanent records of each case.

An adjuvant procedure done to alleviate pelvic pain has been suggested at laser laparoscopy [38].Termed "laser neurectomy," the procedure is mentioned here only in the context of great caution. No controlled trials have evaluated the efficacy of laser neurectomy. Thus, it must continue to be considered an experimental procedure.

The argon laser has been used laparoscopically in rabbits [40] and a small group of women [41] by Keye. The technique involves passing a 0.6 mm flexible quartz fiber through a second-puncture laparoscopic instrument with a steerable tip. Contact with each endometriotic implant is required prior to firing the argon laser. The argon laser is selectively absorbed by the hemoglobin of endometriosis implants, making it potentially safer to deliver to the planned impact site under laparoscopic guidance than carbon dioxide laser laparoscopy. These preliminary results suggest that the argon laser is safe, effective, and easy to use laparoscopically. It lacks the versatility of the carbon dioxide laser because of the argon laser's color-dependency and backscatter. Thus, the use of the argon laser may be limited to photocoagulation of pigmented lesions at laparoscopy or laparotomy.

The Nd:YAG laser has a delivery system similar to that of the argon but with a greater depth of tissue penetration [42]. Preliminary work has demonstrated that visible implants of endometriosis can be coagulated using the Nd:YAG laser. However, the depth of tissue destruction to 3–4 mm mandates extreme caution by the surgeon. As with the argon laser, the surgeon must use special protective lenses because of the hazards of backscatter [33].

To summarize this section, laparoscopic therapy for endometriosis appears to be safe and efficacious, and offers the considerable advantage of shorter recuperative time to the patient. However, there is no area in the clinical study of infertility more flawed by methodologic problems than the applications of laparoscopic surgery [43]. Laparoscopic treatment studies are typically without controls. No effort is made to assess the contribution of treatment-independent conceptions to the "successes" of laparoscopic surgery [44]. When two treatment methods are called similarly successful, there is no analysis of the probability of missing an important therapeutic improvement because of small sample size—the so-called Beta, or Type II error [45]. Finally, the validity in generalizing the excellent results of a few exceptionally dextrous laparoscopic surgeons [21,33,46] to all gynecologists should be questioned. DeCherney, in the same article where he predicts the demise of laparotomy for pelvic reconstructive surgery, makes the observation that "Trying new techniques is alluring; after a brief interval, one believes he is more effective than he is" [16].

CONSERVATIVE SURGERY FOR ENDOMETRIOSIS AT LAPAROTOMY (CSEL)

The indications for CSEL, as graphically demonstrated in Figure 1, include: 1) The persistence of symptoms, including infertility, after suitable trials of expectant, medical, or laparoscopic surgical therapy, 2) Severe endometriosis, or dense adhesions, making laparoscopic surgery difficult and hazardous, 3) The presence of concomitant impediments to fertility that are best treated at laparotomy, e.g., large leiomyomata uteri, 4) The request of the individual patient, who because of age, duration of infertility, or career goals may request the most definitive treatment available, which continues to be CSEL at this time, and 5) A desire by the woman with pelvic pain to avoid hysterectomy even though she has completed her childbearing.

Following laparoscopic diagnosis and staging of endometriosis, and in the presence of indication(s) for CSEL, laparotomy may be performed immediately or delayed for 4 to 12 weeks. Immediate laparotomy offers the advantages of a single anesthetic and a single hospitalization. During preoperative counseling of the couple, the option of immediate versus delayed laparotomy should be discussed; in our experience, 90% of women choose immediate surgery [47]. There is no discernible difference between immediate and delayed laparotomy in terms of complications or pregnancy rates. Although the patient often will express her preference of immediate vs. delayed laparotomy, the surgeon has the responsibility of interpreting that preference based on the operative findings. Should laparoscopy reveal posterior cul-de-sac obliteration, gastrointestinal endometriosis, or extensive disease, the surgeon should consider postponing the procedure and prescribe 2 to 6 months of danazol to better prepare the pelvis for an extensive surgical procedure [48]. In most cases, however, experienced surgeons can effectively manage severe disease without preoperative medical therapy. Preoperative mechanical and antibiotic bowel preparation will reduce complications in the patient who requires a gastrointestinal procedure.

Following induction of anesthesia, pelvic examination is gently performed to detect pelvic masses that may affect the choice of abdominal incision. The cervix is gradually dilated if this has not been carried out at a recent laparoscopic procedure. Similarly, hysteroscopy can be performed if there is a suspicion of uterine anomaly, leiomyomata, endometrial or endocervical polyp, or intrauterine adhesions. A No. 8 pediatric Foley catheter is inserted into the uterine cavity to permit intraoperative chromopertubation.

The patient is prepped and draped in the dorsal supine position. A low transverse incision usually provides adequate exposure; vertical incisions can be used when the woman has a previous vertical scar, or is obese with a narrow pelvis. Gentle handling of tissues throughout the procedure is imperative. The incision edges are draped with moistened laparotomy packs to prevent blood and tissue products from entering the peritoneal cavity. Surgeons should rinse all powder from their gloves prior to entering the peritoneal cavity. The upper abdomen is manually explored, and any omental or bowel adhesions are lysed with meticulous attention to hemostasis. A self-retaining retractor is placed over the moistened wound edge packs; care is taken that the retractor is not resting on the psoas muscle, because of the risk of femoral neuropathy [49]. The bowel is packed away anatomically and atraumatically, avoiding abrasion of the internal genitalia. Grasping instruments and sponge sticks are not used in the pelvis in conservative procedures; gentle retraction with fingers or Teflon-coated malleable retractors is preferable. All pelvic organs are kept moist with intermittent irrigation with lactated Ringer's solution containing 5,000 units of heparin and 40 mg dexamethasone per liter warmed to body temperature [50,51]. Operative loupes of 2.5X magnification are used in many cases. The operative microscope is rarely, if ever, needed for CSEL, as has been recommended [31].

The pelvis is inspected; a stay suture may be placed at the junction of the uterosacral ligaments and the cervix to afford mobility of the uterus without the use of clamps. If the insertion of the uterosacral ligaments is inaccessible, a stay suture may be placed at a higher site on the uterine fundus.

Presacral neurectomy (PSN) remains a useful procedure that is indicated when the patient treated at CSEL complains of central pelvic pain (cf. references 52,53,57). PSN is efficacious in the relief of pain; two early reports claimed proportions of pain relief between 75% and 100% [54,55]. Puolukka et al. [56] reported an increase in pain relief from 80% to 90% when presacral neurectomy was added to complete resection of endometriosis. There is a consensus that presacral neurectomy is a useful palliative procedure in the woman who desires preservation of her fertility potential and complains of central pelvic pain. In our experience, PSN is always performed as a component operation when central pelvic pain accompanies endometriosis.

The effect of PSN on pregnancy rates in infertile women is less clear than its relief of pain. Spangler et al. [58] reported improved pregnancy rates in women treated with PSN at conservative surgery for endometriosis (62%) when compared to CSEL without PSN (44%). However, Polan and De-Cherney [57] found no improvement in pregnancy rates. Most surgeons feel that there is no reliably predictable effect of PSN on pregnancy rates.

Review of the relevant clinical anatomy is useful prior to discussion of operative technique of presacral neurectomy [52,53,59–61]. The lumbar and lower thoracic sympathetic ganglia and the superior, middle, and inferior hypogastric plexuses constitute the sensory pathways from the pelvic organs. Pain impulses from the cervix, uterine fundus, and proximal fallopian tubes pass through afferent fibers that accompany sympathetic nerves into the spinal cord at segments T10, T11, T12, and L1. The fibers merge into the uterine plexus, then the paracervical plexus of Frankenhausen at the base of the uterosacral ligaments. The afferents are carried through the uterosacral ligaments to the sacrum, ascending through the inferior, middle, and superior hypogastric plexuses, and finally the lumbar and lower thoracic sympathetic chain. These sensory nerves are special visceral afferents, independent of the autonomic nervous system.

The superior hypogastric plexus, the anatomically correct name of the presacral nerve, lies in a bed of loose areolar tissue overlying the bodies of the fourth and fifth lumbar vertebrae. It is commonly formed from two or three incompletely fused nerve trunks and may be dispersed in the connective tissue in more than one layer. Twenty percent of patients have complete nerve fusion, forming a single presacral nerve [60]. The middle sacral artery and vein lie in the midline situated between the superior hypogastric plexus and the vertebral periosteum. Other vascular relations include the aorta and vena cava superiorly, a plexus of veins inferiorly in the hollow of the pelvis, the inferior mesenteric vessels to the left, and the right common iliac vessels to the right. The ureters converge on the midline as they exit the pelvis; typically they are found 2–4 cm lateral to the middle sacral vessels. The ureters *must* be clearly identified prior to resection of the presacral nerve.

The technical aspects of presacral neurectomy are straightforward if the anatomic limits of the dissection are kept in mind and the surgeon does not stray beyond them [59]. A 4–5 cm incision is made in the parietal peritoneum over the sacral promontory, and held open with four to six stay sutures. The nerve is dissected from the right margin to the left, with the margins of dissection extending from the right ureter to the left inferior mesenteric artery and vein in the base of the sigmoid mesocolon. Dissection is then carried posterior to the sacral periosteum. The hollow of the sacrum is not entered because of the presence of veins that may cause troublesome bleeding. When the periosteum is reached, a plexus is bluntly dissected off the periosteum, and is divided and ligated with silk sutures. A 2–4 cm segment of nerve tissue is submitted for pathologic examination. Once hemostasis is assured, the peritoneal defect is closed with running 4-0 absorbable suture.

The middle sacral vessels merit special attention owing to their constant variation. In most women, the vessels can be left intact, as dissection of the nerve is anterior to them. However, if bleeding from these vessels occurs, they must be ligated, often requiring that they be suture ligated to the periosteum using 4-0 suture.

Repeat presacral neurectomy should not be performed. Fibrosis and distortion within the retroperitoneal space will further complicate a second attempt at PSN.

Operative and postoperative complications are more common when dissection is carried out from pelvic sidewall to pelvic sidewall, significantly more extensive than the recommended technique. Today, there is little risk of major hemorrhage or significant bowel or bladder dysfunction. However, the rare complication is a serious one; our series of 488 presacral neurectomies has been complicated by ligation and resection of the right ureter in one case and nicking the side of the ureter in another. Histologic inspection of the resected tissue is mandatory, as evidence of ureteric injury may be present in the specimen. Due to the location of the injury high on the sacrum, the preferred technique for repair is a transureteroureterostomy (TUU) performed by an experienced urologic surgeon [70].

Following presacral neurectomy, the surgeon destroys as many of the endometriotic foci as possible in a systematic fashion. The microscope is preferred by some [31]; we use 2.5X to 3.5X operating loupes for magnification. At least one plaque should be excised to histologically confirm the diagnosis. Otherwise, superficial implants are best electrocoagulated or vaporized using the hand-held laser. Sharp dissection is preferred around the colon and ureter. Reperitonealization of surgical defects is performed with running 4-0 or finer absorbable sutures. Large defects can be closed with a free peritoneal graft in preference to an omental graft, or fixation of the round ligaments over some uterine raw areas. Uterosacral ligament plication affords excellent reperitonealization of a raw posterior cul-de-sac and lifts retroverted uteri anteriorly. Care must be taken to avoid plicating the ligaments too far posteriorly; if the space between the plicated ligaments and rectosigmoid is too small, small bowel can herniate into the space, with entrapment resulting in small bowel obstruction.

The extent of ovarian disease may vary from superficial pinpoint lesions to invasive endometriomas that compromise ovarian blood supply. Superficial lesions are fulgurated with cautery or vaporized with laser. Deeper endometriomas may be resected in wedge fashion, "shelled out," or unroofed with subsequent fulguration/vaporization of residual capsule lining. The goals of any ovarian operation are preservation of blood supply to the normal ovarian tissue, complete removal of endometriosis, and plastic closure of the ovarian cortex.

Ovarian endometriosis is typically bilateral, with a statistically greater likelihood of being found on the left ovary, and a greater likelihood of being more severe on the left side. If one adnexa is severely diseased, whereas the contralateral adnexa is spared, unilateral salpingo-oophorectomy has been shown to not adversely affect postoperative pregnancy rates while decreasing reoperation rates [62]. This maneuver is particularly important in the woman with unilateral adnexal pain, which correlates with the more diseased adnexa in most cases.

The adnexal component of the operation is completed with assessment of tubal patency. All peritubular and periovarian adhesions are lysed. Chromopertubation is performed with the previously placed intrauterine Foley, and results carefully recorded in the operative record. Reperitonealization of the areas around the adnexa is individualized. Extensive peritoneal disease requires resection in most cases; primary closure is the treatment of choice if adjacent peritoneum is mobile. If it is not mobile, consideration should be given to use of a free peritoneal graft. The ovaries may be kept out of a raw cul-de-sac by uterosacral ligament plication. Shortening of the uteroovarian ligaments may also be of advantage in elevating the ovary from the cul-de-sac as well. However, as advances are made in transvaginal ultrasonographically guided ovum aspiration, deeper cul-de-sac positions of the ovaries are proving preferable should be patient ultimately require in vitro fertilization.

The uterosacral ligaments are resected only if affected by invasive endometriosis. The resulting defect is closed with absorbable 4-0 suture, with concomitant plication of the ligament to the back of the uterus with 3-0 permanent suture.

Authors differ as to the role of routine appendectomy at the time of CSEL. Occult appendiceal endometriosis occurs in 3% of women with pelvic endometriosis [63]. It is our opinion that appendectomy should be performed only if the appendix appears diseased.

Ten to 15% of endometriosis patients will harbor significant gastrointestinal foci of the disease. Most lesions are superficial and may be destroyed by electrocautery/laser or sharply excised. Nodules invading the bowel wall must be excised. The unusual case of transmural disease is best treated by segmental resection and primary anastomosis. Any patient with severe endometriosis, particularly with rectal symptoms or barium enema/colonoscopic evidence of gastrointestinal involvement, should undergo CSEL with the benefit of a standard mechanical and antibiotic bowel preparation.

Superficial peritoneal disease of the anterior cul-de-sac can be cauterized/vaporized. Invasive nodules of the bladder should be excised with layered closure of the bladder wall to achieve a watertight closure.

Prior to closure of the abdomen, hemostasis is verified and the pelvis is copiously irrigated. Intraperitoneal instillation of 100–200 cc of high molecular weight dextran (Hyskon) is utilized in an attempt to reduce the extent of postoperative adhesions. Perioperative administration of antibiotics is routine.

Short-interval, second-look laparoscopy has become the standard of care following laparotomy for pelvic adhesive disease [22,23]. Our preliminary use of second-look laparoscopy [24] demonstrates it to be a safe method in patients treated by CSEL as well. Ongoing studies will evaluate pregnancy and reoperation rates following adhesiolysis in the immediate postoperative period in the CSEL patient.

CSEL is associated with few operative complications [64]. Subsequent pregnancy rates range in the literature from 13% to 94%. A recent review by Olive [65] which includes 1,635 patients treated by CSEL from 1963 to 1985, demonstrates an overall 54% pregnancy rate. He then summarizes the overall pregnancy rates by classification of disease; mild endometriosis treated by CSEL (CSEL is rarely indicated for mild disease today) is associated with a 62% pregnancy rate in 278 patients, moderate with a 52% pregnancy rate in 363 patients, and severe with a 40% overall pregnancy rate in 382 patients. Olive appropriately points out that most of these studies presented their data in terms of crude pregnancy rates; we hope that future studies will utilize the statistically more desirable techniques of life table analysis and monthly fecundity rates [13].

Our most recent data [66] on over 400 patients treated by CSEL is presented in Table II. The observed pregnancy rates fit well with Olive's literature review. Life table projections of expected pregnancy rates compensate for patients lost to follow-up and those currently attempting conception.

Annual rates of recurrence are presented in Table III. Cumulative reoperation rates are 13% at 3 years and 32% at 5 years. Most clinical studies of endometriosis fail to describe recurrence or reoperation rates; it is hoped with longer periods of follow-up that the natural history of recurrent endometriosis will be better described [12,66].

Perioperative Danazol Therapy

Perioperative medical suppression is based on the thinking that surgical therapy is at best a "debulking" operation. Preoperative danazol is aimed at improving the pelvic environment for surgery; postoperative danazol is

TABLE II. Predicted and Observed Pregnancy Rates by Grade of Severity Following Conservative Surgery for Endometriosis at Laparotomy

Acosta classification	Predicted pregnancy rate[a] (%)	Observed pregnancy rate[b] (%)
Mild (N = 136)	81	57 (78/136)
Moderate (N = 69)	87	54 (37/69)
Severe (N = 172)	65	36 (63/172)

[a]Life table projection for 10 years of follow-up.
[b]Observed pregnancy rates regardless of length of follow-up.

TABLE III. Annual Rates of Recurrence and Reoperation in 423 Patients Treated With Conservative Operation for Endometriosis at Laparotomy

	Postoperative year								
	1	2	3	4	5	6	7	8	9+
Patients followed	423	272	170	111	77	51	30	22	12
No reoperation	417	254	161	105	67	45	28	18	11
Reoperation (N = 62)	6 (1.4%)	18 (6.6%)	9 (5.3%)	6 (5.4%)	10 (13.0%)	6 (11.8%)	2 (6.7%)	4 (18.2)	1 (8.3%)
Recurrence at reoperation (N = 41)	4 (0.9%)	13 (4.8%)	6 (3.5%)	3 (2.7%)	5 (6.5%)	4 (7.8%)	2 (6.7%)	3 (13.6%)	1 (8.3%)

prescribed to suppress any residual gross or microscopic nests of endometriosis. We have continued our study of postoperative danazol [67,68]; we continue to find that immediate postoperative danazol significantly improves pregnancy rates in women with severe endometriosis when compared to CSEL alone based on 18-month pregnancy rates of 70% vs. 40%, respectively. The issue of pre-versus postoperative danazol will need to be settled by a prospective comparative trial.

Complete Operations

Hysterectomy is indicated for women with significant endometriosis refractory to more conservative medical and surgical treatment (see Fig. 1). It is also one of the first-line treatments for symptomatic women who have completed their childbearing.

A conservative approach is warranted in regard to ovarian preservation. If the blood supply to the ovaries is intact and the ovaries are not diseased or compromised by adhesions, then preservation is indicated. Should oophorectomy be necessary, exogenous estrogen/progestogen replacement may be ordered. The risk of recurrent endometriosis is low (3% at 5 years) and is not affected by either ovarian preservation or appropriate-dose hormone replacement therapy [69]. Premarin is prescribed at 0.625–.9 mg per day on days 1–28 of each cycle. Adjustments in the cycle and dosage are dependent upon patient tolerance.

REFERENCES

1. Jones HW Jr: The impact of in vitro fertilization on the practice of gynecology and obstetrics. Int J Fertil 31(2):99, 1986.
2. Buttram VC Jr: Evaluation of the revised American Fertility Society classification of endometriosis. Fertil Steril 43:347, 1985.
3. American Fertility Society: Revised American Fertility Society classification of endometriosis. Fertil Steril 43:347, 1985.
4. Schmidt CL: Endometriosis: a reappraisal of pathogenesis and treatment. Fertil Steril 44:157, 1985.
5. Wheeler JM, Malinak LR: Application of computerized pelvic mapping to the conservative surgical treatment of endometriosis: analysis of anatomic areas in relation to postoperative pregnancy. Presented at the Forty-first Annual Meeting of the American Fertility Society, Chicago, Illinois, September 30, 1985 (abstract).
6. Seibel MM: Minimal pelvic endometriosis and infertility. Semin Reprod Endocrinol 3(4):307, 1985.
7. Barbieri RL, Ryan KJ: Medical therapy for endometriosis: endocrine pharmacology. Semin Reprod Endocrinol 3(4):339, 1985.
8. Meldrum DR: Management of endometriosis with gonadotropin releasing hormone agonists. Fertil Steril 44:581, 1985.

9. Schrioch E, Monroe SE, Henzl J, Jaffe RB: Treatment of endometriosis with a potent agonist of gonadotropin-releasing hormone (nafarelin). Fertil Steril 44:583, 1985.
10. Buttram VC Jr: Cyclic use of combination oral contraceptives and the severity of endometriosis. Fertil Steril 31:347, 1979.
11. Cramer D et al.: Association of endometriosis with oral contraceptive use. Presented at the 42nd Annual Meeting of the American Fertility Society, Toronto, October 2, 1986 (abstract).
12. Wheeler JM, Malinak LR: Recurrent endometriosis: incidence, management, and prognosis. Fertil Steril 39:656, 1983.
13. Wheeler JM, Meacham RB, Curran MLC, Malinak LR: Conservative surgery for endometriosis: life table analysis of prognostic factors for pregnancy and reoperation. Presented at the Annual District VII Meeting, American College of Obstetricians and Gynecologists, Houston, October, 1983 (abstract).
14. Chilik C, Rosenwaks F: Endometriosis and in vitro fertilization. Semin Reprod Endocrinol 3:377,1985.
15. Corson SL: Use of the laparoscope in the infertile patient. Fertil Steril 32(4):359, 1979.
16. DeCherney AH: The leader of the band is tired. . . . Fertil Steril 44:299, 1985.
17. Dodge ST, Pumphrey RS, Miyazala K: Peritoneal endometriosis in women requesting reversal of sterilization. Fertil Steril 45:774, 1986.
18. Murphy AA, Green WR, Dobbie D, dela Cruz ZC, Rock JA: Unsuspected endometriosis documented by scanning electron microscopy in visually normal peritoneum. Fertil Steril 46:522,1986.
19. Daniell J: Laser laparoscopy for endometriosis. Colp Gynecol Laser Surg 1:185, 1984.
20. Daniell J: Operative laparoscopy for endometriosis. Semin Reprod Endocrinol 3(4):353, 1985.
21. Nezhat C, Crowgey SR, Garrison CP: Surgical treatment of endometriosis via laser laparoscopy. Fertil Steril 45(6):778, 1986.
22. Daniel JF, Pittaway DE: Short interval second-look laparoscopy after infertility surgery: a preliminary report. J Reprod Med 28:281, 1983.
23. Diamond MP, Daniell JF, Martin DC, Feste J, Vaughn WK, McLaughlin DS: Tubal patency and pelvic adhesions at early second-look laparoscopy following intraabdominal use of the carbon dioxide laser: initial report of the intraabdominal laser study group. Fertil Steril 42(5):717, 1984.
24. Wheeler JM, Simolke G, Malinak LR: Second look laparoscopy following conservative surgical therapy at laparotomy for endometriosis. Presented at the Society of Gynecologic Surgeons, New Orleans, March, 1986 (abstract).
25. Frangenheim H: "Laparoscopy and Culdoscopy in Gynecology." London: Buttersworth, p 35, 1972.
26. Semm, K: "Atlas of Gynecologic Laparoscopy and Hysteroscopy." Philadelphia: WB Saunders Co., p 232, 1975.
27. Eward, RD: Cauterization of Stage I and II endometriosis and resulting pregnancy rate. In Phillips JM, Downey CA (eds.): "Endoscopy and Gynecology." Santa Fe Springs, CA: American Association of Gynecologic Laparoscopists, p 271, 1978.
28. Hasson HM: Electrocoagulation of pelvic endometriosis lesions with laparoscopic control. Am J Obstet Gynecol 132:115, 1979.
29. Sulewski JM, Crucia FD, Brenitskey C: The treatment of endometriosis at laparoscopy for infertility. Am J Obstet Gynecol 128:128, 1980.
30. Daniell JF, Christiansen C: Combined laparoscopic surgery and danazol therapy for pelvic endometriosis. Fertil Steril 35:521, 1981.

31. Bellina JH: Gynecology and the laser. Contemp Obstet Gynecol 4:24, 1974.
32. Pittaway DE, Matson WS, Daniell JF: A comparison of the CO2 laser and electrocautery on postoperative adhesion formation in rabbits. Fertil Steril 40:366, 1983.
33. Daniell JF: The role of lasers in infertility surgery. Fertil Steril 42 (6):815, 1984.
34. Grunert GM, Franklin RR: What's new: the laser in gynecologic fertility survey. Texas Med 79:43, 1983.
35. Bruhat M, Mage C, Manhes M: Use of the CO2 laser via laparoscopy. In Laser Surgery III, Proceedings of the Third International Society for Laser Surgery, EAI Kaplan, Tel Aviv, p. 275, 1979.
36. Daniell JF, Pittaway DE: Use of the CO2 laser in laparoscopic surgery: initial experience with the second puncture technique. Infertility 5:15, 1982.
37. Kelly RW, Roberts DK: CO2 laser laparoscopy: potential alternative to danazol in the treatment of Stage I and II endometriosis. J Reprod Med 28:638, 1980.
38. Feste JR: Laser laparoscopy: a new modality, Lasers Surg Med 3:170, 1983.
39. Martin DC: CO2 laser laparoscopy for the treatment of endometriosis associated with infertility. J Reprod Med 30:409, 1985.
40. Keye WR Jr. Matson GA, Dixon J: The use of the argon laser in the treatment of experimental endometriosis. Fertil Steril 39:26, 1983.
41. Keye WR Jr, Dixon J: Photocoagulation of endometriosis by the argon laser through the laparoscope. Obstet Gynecol 62:383, 1983.
42. Lamano JM: Photocoagulation of ealry pelvic endometriosis by the Nd:YAG laser through the laparoscope. J Reprod Med 30 (2):77, 1985.
43. Olive DL: Analysis of clinical fertility trials: a methodologic review. Fertil Steril 45(2):157, 1986.
44. Collins JA, Wrixon W, Jones, LB, Wilson EH: Treatment - independent pregnancy among infertile couples, N Engl J Med 309(20):1201, 1983.
45. Freiman JA, Chalmer TC, Smith H Jr. Kuebler RR: The importance of Beta, the Type II error and sample size in the design and interpretation of the randomized control trial. N Engl J Med 299:690, 1978.
46. Reich H, McGlynn F: Treatment of ovarian endometriosis using laparoscopic surgical techniques. J Reprod Med 31 (7):577, 1986.
47. Maccato MLK, Wheeler JM, Malinak LR: The timing of laparoscopy to laparotomy in the surgical treatment of female infertility. Presented to the American College of Obstetricians and Gynecologists, Washington, D.C., May, 1985 (abstract).
48. Buttram VC Jr, Reiter RC, Ward S: Treatment of endometriosis with danazol: report of a 6-year prospective study. Fertil Steril 43:353, 1985.
49. Hassan AA, Reiff RH, Fayez JA: Femoral neuropathy following microsurgical tuboplasty. Fertil Steril 45(6):889, 1986.
50. Malinak LR: Infertility and endometriosis: operative technique, clinical staging and prognosis, Clin Obstet Gynecol 23:925, 1980.
51. Buttram VC Jr: Surgical therapy of endometriosis in the infertile female: a modified approach. Fertil Steril 32:635, 1979.
52. Malinak LR, Wheeler JM: Presacral neurectomy. In C-R Garcia "Current Therapy in Surgical Gynecology." (ed): In Press.
53. Malinak LR: Operative management of pelvic pain. In (ed): "Gynecology and Obstetrics." Vol. 1. Chapter 78. Sciarra JJ Philadelphia: Harper & Row, p 1, 1984.
54. Greenhill JP: Sympathectomy for the relief of pain in women. J Mt Sinai Hosp 14:363, 1947.

55. Black WT Jr: Use of presacral neurectomy in the treatment of dysmenorrhea. Am J Obstet Gynecol 89:16, 1914.
56. Puolakka J, Kouppila A, Ronnberg C: Results in the operative treatment of pelvic endometriosis. Acta Obstet Gynecol Scand 59:429, 1980.
57. Polan ML, DeCherney AH: Presacral neurectomy for pelvic pain in infertility. Fertil Steril 34:557, 1980.
58. Spangler DB, Jones GS Jones HW Jr: Infertility due to endometriosis. Am J Obstet Gynecol 109:850, 1971.
59. Curtis AH, Anson BJ, Ashly FL, Jones T: The anatomy of the pelvic autonomic nerves in relation to gynecology. Surg Gynecol Obstet 75:743, 1942.
60. Whorton LR: Presacral neurectomy. In Mattingly RE (ed): "TeLinde's Operative Gynecology," 5th ed. Philadelphia: Lippincott, p 253, 1977.
61. Kistner RW, Patton GW Jr: Presacral neurectomy and uterine suspension. In "Atlas of Infertility Surgery" Boston: Little, Brown, p 189, 1975.
62. Wheeler JM, Maccato ML, Malinak LR: The role of unilateral salpingo-oophorectomy in the conservative surgical treatment of endometriosis. Presented at the 41st Annual Meeting of the American Fertility Society, Chicago, September 30, 1985 (abstract).
63. Buttram VC Jr, Betts JW: Endometriosis. Curr Prob Obstet Gynecol 2:1, 1979.
64. Wheeler JM, Meacham RB, Malinak LR: Complications of infertility surgery (submitted).
65. Olive DL: Endometriosis. In DeCherney AH (ed): "Reproductive Failure." New York: Churchill-Livingston, p 183, 1986.
66. Malinak LR, Wheeler JM: Association of endometriosis with spontaneous abortion, prognosis for pregnancy, and risk for recurrence. Semin Reprod Endocrinol 3(4):361, 1985.
67. Wheeler JM, Malinak LR: Postoperative danazol therapy in infertility patients with severe endometriosis. Fertil Steril 36:460, 1981.
68. Wheeler JM, Maccato ML, Malinak LR: Postoperative danazol: pregnancy rates in women with endometriosis treated by combined surgical therapy/immediate postoperative danazol. Presented at the 41st Annual Meeting of the American Fertility Society, Chicago, September 30, 1985 (abstract).
69. Wheeler JM, Christie R, Young RL, Buttram VC Jr, Malinak LR: Endometriosis at hysterectomy: incidence of recurrence according to ovarian preservation vs estrogen replacement. Presented to the Annual Clinical Meeting of the American College of Obstetricians and Gynecologists, Washington, DC, May, 1985 (abstract).

Endometriosis, pages 161–172

Chapter 9
Endometriosis in Adolescents

Joseph S. Sanfilippo, M.D.

Department of Obstetrics and Gynecology, University of Louisville School of Medicine, Louisville, Kentucky 40292

INTRODUCTION

Endometriosis is considered to be a disease found in women usually in their twenties or thirties who have postponed childbearing, and is not considered to be a disorder commonly found in teenagers. This should be of significant concern to the clinician, as endometriosis can affect a young woman's fertility potential. Symptoms of endometriosis must first be differentiated from other causes of pelvic pain such as gastrointestinal problems, genitourinary complaints, and infections of the reproductive tract (Table I). Clinical presentation and treatment of endometriosis is similar for adolescents and older women alike. However, although adolescents are seldom concerned with fertility, they should be questioned extensively about associated symptoms and their interest in future fertility. In most cases, treatment for adolescents should be directed toward forestalling the progress of the disease.

INCIDENCE OF ADOLESCENT ENDOMETRIOSIS

Although endometriosis has been a recognized disorder for years [1,2], the exact rate of occurrence of endometriosis in adolescents is difficult to establish. However, prevalence of this disorder in young women may not differ greatly from that in older women. Ranney [3] has suggested that between 4% and 17% of all menstruating women have pelvic endometriosis. The incidence, in part, depends upon the patient population. In the adolescent age group, Meigs [4] reported a 6% incidence at laparoscopy. In adolescents presenting with chronic pelvic pain, Goldstein et al. [5] reported 47% with endometriosis.

TABLE I. Causes of Acute and Chronic Abdominal Pain in the Adolescent

Hematometra	Meckel's diverticulum with abscess
Intussusception	Ulcerative colitis
Peritonitis	Constipation
Perforation of a viscus	Urinary tract infection
Urinary calculus	Porphyria
Hematosalpinx	Sickle cell anemia
Pelvic inflammatory disease	Mesenteric lymphadenitis
Imperforate hymen	Hydronephrosis
Vaginal septum	Liver cysts (oral contraceptive related)
Blind pouch of the vagina with hematometra	Bowel obstruction
Ectopic pregnancy	Splenomegaly
Chronic pancreatitis	Neuroblastoma
Regional enteritis	Urachal cysts

Reprinted with permission: Lavery JP, Sanfilippo JS (eds): "Pediatric and Adolescent Obstetrics and Gynecology." New York: Springer Verlag, 1985.

Endometriosis is thought to occur rarely in indigent women and in young black women. Racial differences in the prevalence of the disease are unlikely. Chatman [6] found endometriosis in 21% of black women undergoing laparoscopy for various symptoms. Of those patients with endometriosis, 12.5% were 15–19 years of age. Why the incidence appears to be less in the lower socioeconomic class is not thought to be related to disease immunity but rather to malnutrition, poor living conditions, high rates of pelvic inflammatory disease, early marriage, early and frequent childbearing, and inability to obtain medical attention [7]. Adolescents at increased risk for endometriosis are those with genital tract anomalies [5,8,9].

Table II is a review of publications addressing endometriosis in the adolescent [4,5,8,10–24].

DEVELOPMENT OF ENDOMETRIOSIS

Fallon believes development of endometriosis requires 5 or more years of menstrual cycles with premenstrual ovulation [10]. The mean interval between menarche and diagnosis of endometriosis has been calculated at 4.5 years. The youngest patient ever reported to have endometriosis was 10.5 years of age [5]. She had experienced menarche 5 months earlier. Although menarche is thought by many to precede the development of endometriosis, Whitehouse [25] reported endometriosis in a 22-year-old female with primary amenorrhea. Similarly, Seitz [26] reported endometriomas in a 21-year-old with primary amenorrhea. While we know that older teens are more likely to seek gynecological care than are younger adolescents, we must also realize that the disease can and does exist in the preteen and early teenager.

TABLE II. Endometriosis in Adolescents

Meigs [4]	Endometrial cysts in 13- to 19-year-old adolescents.
Goldstein et al. [5]	Endometriosis was found in 74 (52%) of 140 adolescents with pelvic pain; 11% had genital anomalies.
Schifrin et al. [8]	Fifteen cases of endometriosis in patients 12 to 20 years old and presenting with epigastric, lower quadrant abdominal pain, or dysmenorrhea. There was an associated increased incidence of GI and GU anomalies.
Fallon [10]	Four percent of teenage females (9 of 225) had endometriosis. Four of the 9 had endometriosis at the time of preoperative diagnosis of acute appendicitis.
Derryberry and Bonney [11]	Endometrioma in a 15-year-old black female with a normal vagina, introitus, and a stenotic cervical isthmus.
Bullock et al. [12]	Symptomatic endometriosis in teenagers. Wilford Hall, USAF Medical Center, four cases, 17 to 19 years old.
Hanton et al. [13]	Sixty-eight young patients (62-menarche, 5 to 10 years before the diagnosis, and 6-congenital obstruction to menstrual flow) in a 30-year review of cases at the Mayo Clinic.
Hanton et al. [14]	Case report of endometriosis associated with complete or partial obstruction of menstrual egress.
Moore et al. [15]	Seven of 127 patients with ovarian masses had endometriosis; age range: birth to 17.
Bruser [16]	Appendectomy with inability to relieve symptoms. Twelve patients, 19 to 31 years old. Subsequently each was found to have endometriosis.
Depp and Pope [17]	Of 233 patients between 10 and 19, 2.3% had endometriosis.
TeLinde [18]	Of 8,789 pelvic laparotomies, 1.2% had microscopically diagnosed endometriosis within 10 years of menarche.
Sutton [19]	A 14-year-old with imperforate hymen, hematocolpos, hematometra (bilateral hematosalpinges, and peritoneal implants).
Sutton [20]	Etiological factors in endometriosis—case of reflux menstruation with a bicornuate uterus. Intense distended left horn.
McDonald [21]	Endometriosis associated with didelphic uterus.
King [22]	Metastatic endometriosis in abdominal scars of a 17-year-old female. Pain and tenderness with right lower quadrant abdominal pain noted with a preoperative diagnosis of acute appendicitis.
Mittal et al. [23]	Endometriosis of the appendix, presenting as acute appendicitis. Patients were 14 to 62 years old. Forty percent (20 of 50) incidence of GI tract involvement with endometriosis.
Chatman and Ward [24]	Endometriosis was found in 65% of 43 black teenagers.

Reprinted with permission: Lavery JP, Sanfilippo JS (eds): "Pediatric and Adolescent Obstetrics and Gynecology." New York: Springer Verlag, 1985.

The exact mechanism of development of endometriosis is not clearly understood. Thus, the current theories of origin apply to adults and to adolescents alike. These theories include: 1) Sampson's theory of retrograde menstruation, 2) Meyer's theory of totipotential cells undergoing metaplasia, 3) hematogenous dissemination, and 4) lymphatic spread. No one theory provides a total answer (see Chapter 2).

A genetic or familial influence on the occurrence of endometriosis has been demonstrated. A polygenic multifactorial mode of inheritance for endometriosis has been reported by Simpson et al. [27], who found a 6.9% rate of endometriosis in first-degree relatives of women with the disease compared with only 1% in control relatives. Thus, endometriosis should be suspected in symptomatic adolescents who have a family history of the disease.

The major distinction between adolescents and older women in the development of endometriosis is its association with anomalies of the reproductive system. Several anomalies associated with the reproductive tract and development of endometriosis have been reported, including imperforate hymen, vaginal septum, hematocolpos, hematometra, uterine anomalies, and associated urinary tract abnormalities such as renal agenesis [8]. Any obstruction of the outflow tract seems to be associated with the formation of endometriosis. Examples of reproductive tract anomalies that may cause endometriosis are presented in Figure 1. In a series reported by Schifrin et al. [8], 6 of 15 endometriosis patients (40%) under age 20 had a genital tract anomaly. Goldstein and coworkers [5] found congenital abnormalities of the reproductive tract in 11% of 74 teenagers with endometriosis.

The clinical course of endometriosis when associated with a reproductive tract abnormality appears to be different from that in which endometriosis is not associated with outflow obstruction. In such cases, when a patent outflow tract is established, reversal of extensive pelvic cavity endometriosis results [9].

Endometriosis has been reported to be associated with mature ovarian teratomas and gliomatosis peritonei in a 10-year-old patient [28]. Endometriosis also has been associated with "smooth muscle metaplasia" [29], hemangiomas [30], and leiomyomas and adenomyosis of the gastrointestinal tract [31] in adolescent girls. In addition, metastatic endometriosis in abdominal scars has been reported [32]. The endometriosis associated with these disorders is likely to be incidental and not specifically related to the disorder.

CLINICAL PRESENTATION

The characteristic symptoms associated with endometriosis are pelvic pain and infertility (see Chapter 3). Since fertility is usually not a concern of

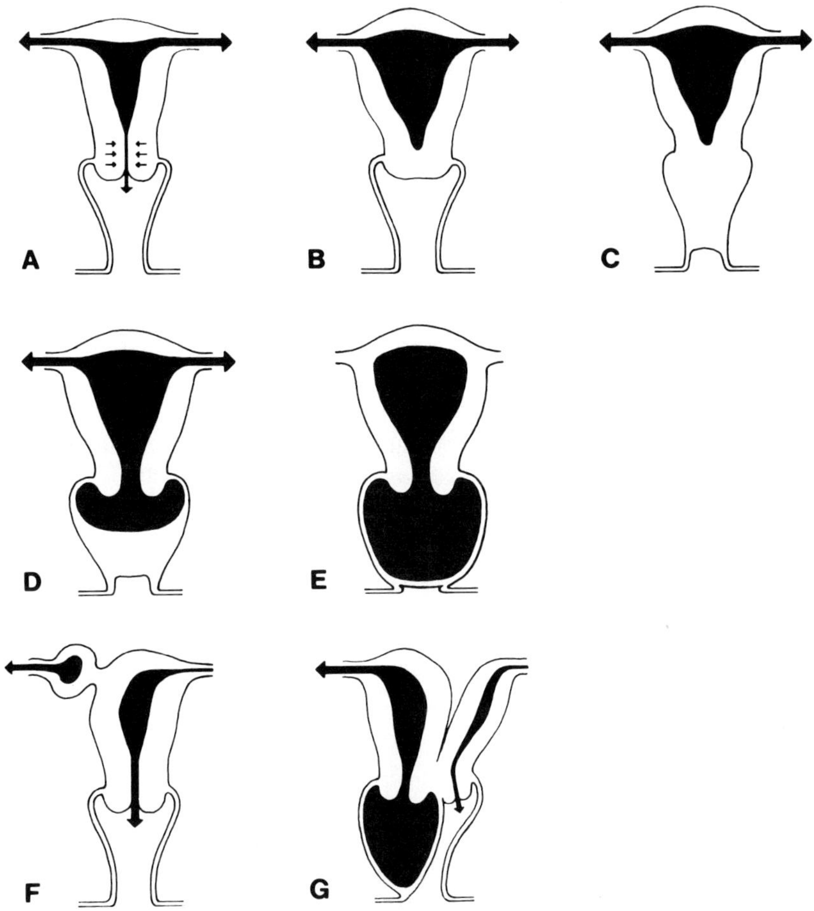

Fig. 1. Anomalies of the reproductive tract that could result in adolescent endometriosis. **A.** Cervical stenosis, **B.** Cervical agenesis, **C.** Vaginal agenesis, **D.** Transverse vaginal septum, **E.** Imperforate hymen, **F.** Rudimentary uterine horn, **G.** Unilateral vaginal obstruction.

theirs, adolescents usually complain of chronic pelvic pain or dysmenorrhea. In a study of teenagers with documented endometriosis, Chatman and Ward [24] found that the most common complaint was dysmenorrhea in 78% of patients, followed by abnormal bleeding in 35%, bowel symptoms in 37%, and dyspareunia in 14%. Similar presenting symptoms were reported by Goldstein et al. [5] in 66 adolescent girls with endometriosis (see Table III). The dysmenorrhea is usually acquired and increases in severity with age.

TABLE III. Presenting Symptoms in 66 Adolescents With Endometriosis [5]

Symptom	Patients No.	Patients %
Pain	66	100
Cyclic	42	64
Acyclic	24	36
Abnormal Bleeding	18	28
Dyspareunia	17	25
Gastrointestinal symptoms	14	21

Reprinted by permission of Elsevier Science Publishing Co., Inc., from Goldstein D et al.: Adolescent Endometriosis. J Adol Heath Care 1: 37, 1980.

The typical presentation is that of dysmenorrhea refractory to nonsteroidal antiinflammatory agents and, in some cases, oral contraceptive therapy. However, although some relief can be obtained with these agents initially, it is usually not long lasting. Furthermore, endometriosis may cause further ovarian dysfunction and abnormal bleeding. Bowel symptoms include rectal pressure, pain on defecation, and urgency, especially during the late luteal and menstrual phases. The high percentage of young patients with bowel symptoms (21–37%) is somewhat surprising, but it emphasizes how endometriosis can progress symptomatically even in adolescents. Dyspareunia is another common form of pelvic pain associated with endometriosis that teenagers may also begin to experience but may be reluctant to report. The dyspareunia is likely related to the presence of tender endometriotic implants in the cul-de-sac.

Preoperative pelvic findings in teenagers with endometriosis are similar to those found in older patients. Chatman and Ward [24] found that tenderness in the cul-de-sac could be elicited in 78% of adolescents with documented endometriosis, and nodularity with tenderness in 36%. Adnexal masses were present in 11% of teenagers. When Goldstein et al. [5] evaluated adolescents with endometriosis, 76% were noted to have pelvic tenderness, 22% cul-de-sac nodularity, and 27% a distinct adnexal mass. Eleven percent of patients had a fixed, retroverted uterus.

Often, the pelvic examination is normal even in patients with endometriosis. In the series by Goldstein and coworkers [5], 17% of young women had a normal examination. These authors emphasized that the examination should be performed during menses or the late luteal phase in order to enhance the pelvic findings.

DIAGNOSIS

A diagnosis of endometriosis is common in adolescents who are experiencing pain. A careful history of symptoms characteristic of endometriosis is helpful in diagnosing this disorder as well as in distinguishing it from other causes of pelvic pain (see Table I).

Pelvic examination in an adolescent may be difficult, and rectal examination may be the only means to evaluate the pelvis for tenderness, nodularity, retrodisplaced uterus, or adnexal masses. Anomalies of the hymen, vagina, and cervix can be detected during pelvic examination, and a search should be made for these and other congenital abnormalities that are more likely to cause adolescent endometriosis. An analgesic cocktail or even general anesthesia may be required for adequate evaluation of the pelvis.

Ultrasonography may be helpful, particularly in adolescents difficult to examine, or when documenting the presence or size of adnexal masses. Ultrasonography can also be used to monitor the size of ovarian cysts in response to therapy. However, endometriomas cannot be distinguished from other pelvic masses by ultrasound, and a persistent mass requires surgical evaluation.

Preoperative evaluation of patients presenting with chronic pelvic pain should also include a complete blood count, urine analysis, cervical cytology, and sedimentation rate. Cervical and urethral cultures, including those for chlamydia, can be performed to identify those patients with acute or chronic inflammatory processes.

Diagnostic laparoscopy is an integral part of the assessment of pelvic pain and diagnosis of endometriosis in adolescent patients. As stated above, in 140 patients between age 10.5 and 19 presenting with chronic pain, Goldstein and associates [5] confirmed endometriosis in 52%. Early endometriosis usually does not appear as the characteristic "blue-black" lesions. Hemorrhagic areas have been noted by Goldstein et al. [5] to be "biopsy proven" endometriosis. Furthermore, 20% of biopsied lesions were not grossly typical of endometriosis. Consequently, the clinician must be aware that early endometriosis may present with a hemorrhagic or petechial appearance.

When endometriosis is evidenced at laparoscopy, the American Fertility Society Revised Classification should be employed, not only to determine the extent of disease but to aid in the choice of therapy (see Chapter 5). Using the Acosta classification, Chatman and Ward [24] reported that in their series of patients, 50% had mild disease, 39% had moderate disease, and 11% had severe disease. A similar distribution was seen by Goldstein et al. [5]. At present, there is no clear correlation between age and severity of disease.

Endometriosis in the adolescent is more likely to be severe when it is associated with outflow obstruction [9].

TREATMENT

For an adolescent who has no immediate interest in fertility, treatment centers primarily on control of pain. When pelvic pain is encountered in an adolescent, nonsteroidal antiinflammatory agents should be prescribed with the initial onset of pain or prior to anticipated pain and continued on a regular basis until the pain has completely subsided. All antiprostaglandins basically inhibit prostaglandin synthesis and/or inhibit prostaglandin binding to its receptors to alleviate dysmenorrhea. For the adolescent with cyclical pelvic pain who does not respond to nonsteroidal antiprostaglandins, the next step is to suppress ovulation with an oral contraceptive. A high-progestin, low-estrogen (35–50 mcg) preparation should be prescribed in the usual cyclical manner. Failure of these primary measures to alleviate symptoms indicates a need for further evaluation.

Diagnosis of endometriosis primarily involves operative assessment of the pelvic organs. Endometriosis is often an unexpected surgical finding in an adolescent, and there are usually questions regarding intraoperative and postoperative management. Prior to scheduling any surgical intervention, the physician should counsel the patient and parent (guardian) about the possible need for intraoperative therapeutic alternatives such as laparoscopic fulguration or laser vaporization of the endometrial foci. Improvement in symptoms is greater when fulguration of implants and lysis of adhesions is performed during laparoscopy than when laparoscopy is performed for diagnosis alone [5]. Rarely, conservative surgery (laparotomy) may be necessary at the same operative setting. Persistent endometriomas should be excised, leaving as much functional ovarian tissue as possible. If a laparotomy is performed, uterine suspension and approximation of the uterosacral ligaments should be considered, particularly when endometriosis is present in the cul-de-sac or partial obliteration of the cul-de-sac has occurred. At this setting, presacral neurectomy may also be considered, especially if pelvic pain is severe. Hemostasis and care with handling of tissues is of primary importance in the prevention of subsequent adhesion formation. Solutions such as 32% dextran 70 (Hyskon®) or Ringers Lactate left in the abdomen postoperatively may also reduce adhesions. Conservative surgical techniques are reviewed in Chapter 8.

The patient should be carefully evaluated for congenital anomalies of the reproductive tract that may obstruct menstrual outflow. The cervix should be probed and/or dilated to assure patency of the cervical canal and to alleviate any element of stenosis. It is important for the clinician to correct obstruction and retrograde menstruation promptly in order to prevent or reverse endometriosis. Vaginal splinting or continued dilations may be required to maintain a patent outflow tract. If these initial measures are unsuccessful, removal of the involved mullerian structures should be considered. A didelphic or rudimentary uterus with unilateral obstruction also can be surgically corrected by lateral anastomosis of the obstructed horn to the unobstructed horn. Details of treatment alternatives for mullerian anomalies are addressed by Jones [33].

Postoperative management of the adolescent patient with endometriosis is a unique challenge. In addition to pain control, the major concern is the preservation of subsequent fertility. Patients interested in fertility usually would be advised to attempt pregnancy as soon as possible. For most teenagers, however, pregnancy in the immediate postoperative period is not an alternative. In these young women, the issue is how to preserve fertility by preventing further progression of the endometriosis. No well-designed studies have been conducted on the treatment of endometriosis in adolescents. The postoperative management of these patients is based on our knowledge of endometriosis, which is inadequate, use of medical therapy, some actions of which are theoretical, and clinical experience, which is anecdotal.

Following laparoscopic or conservative surgery, some form of medical therapy usually is advised to prevent progression of the disease and preserve childbearing function. Not all of these patients will have difficulty achieving pregnancy, but the clinical presumption is that most patients do. In any event, the types of medical therapy for adolescents are the same as for all patients with endometriosis. Medical therapy is reviewed in Chapter 7.

The choice of medication and dosage regimen may differ when childbearing is to be delayed for several years. For example, danazol is frequently used for 3–6 months, but prolonged administration is not advised because it is reported to have adverse effects on steroid enzymatic pathways and plasma lipids [34–37], liver function [34] and thyroid function [38]. Methyltestosterone may cause masculinization. Even LHRH agonists may cause osteoporosis or other side effects of estrogen depletion when administered for prolonged periods.

Most clinicians use one of the following postoperative medical regimens: 1) danazol 400–800 mg daily for 3–6 months with no subsequent therapy, 2) progestin-dominant oral contraceptive therapy continuously for 6–9 months, 3) medroxyprogesterone acetate (i.e., Provera®, the UpJohn Company, Kalamazoo, MI) 20–30 mg daily for 6–9 months, 4) cyclic progestin-dominant oral contraceptives administered indefinitely until childbearing is desired,

5) danazol for 3–6 months followed by cyclic oral contraceptive therapy, and 6) depo-medroxy progesterone acetate (Depo-Provera®, the UpJohn Company, Kalamazoo, MI) 100 mg IM monthly.

Theoretically, progestin-dominant oral contraceptives (e.g., Ovral or LoOvral containing ethinyl estradiol and norgestrel) prevent progression of endometriosis by suppressing endometrial growth and reducing the amount of menstrual reflux, but the therapeutic value of contraceptive steroids given cyclically has never been substantiated [39,40]. However, their theoretical efficacy and relative safety provide impetus for their long-term use in these patients. Finally, medroxyprogesterone acetate in depo form may be the best alternative for adolescents who wish to delay childbearing. Goldstein et al. [5] reported that when compared with danazol and continuous use of oral progestins, depo-medroxyprogesterone acetate was the most effective from the point of side effects and overall symptomatic improvement. Usually, this medication is not used because of significant delays in return of ovarian function (7–9 months) and fertility (approximately 13 months) [41], but it may be appropriate for adolescents in whom delayed childbearing is desired.

Conservative surgery during or following postoperative medical therapy should be performed only for persistent pain associated with endometriosis, subsequent infertility, or endometriosis compromising other organ systems. The symptomatic results of conservative surgery are favorable and may exceed those of operative laparoscopy and medical therapy [5].

COMMENTS

Evaluation of pelvic pain in the adolescent requires a systematic approach. The patient with recurrent lower abdominal pain in a cyclical pattern who has a normal pelvic examination is best treated initially with nonsteroidal antiinflammatory agents, next by oral contraceptive therapy. If these measures fail to alleviate the symptoms, consideration should be given to diagnostic laparoscopy with intraoperative resection of the foci of endometriosis via either bipolar coagulation or laser vaporization. Depending upon postoperative symptoms and reevaluation, ovulation suppression with any of several medical modalities of treatment is in order.

REFERENCES

1. Ebers G: The papyrus ebers-1. Chap.97, p.112 Leipzig 1973; translated by E Bell, B Lewin, and E Munksgaard, Copenhagen: Jnar Munksgaard, 1937.
2. von Rokitansky, Ueber Uterusdausen-Newbildung in Uterus and Ovarial sarcomen. Ztschr d.k.k. Gesell Schd. Aertte zuWien 37:577, 1960.

3. Ranney B: Etiology, prevention and inhibition of endometriosis. Clin Obstet Gynecol 23:875, 1980.
4. Meigs J: Endometriosis. Ann Surg 127:795, 1948.
5. Goldstein D, DeCholnoky C, Emans SJ: Adolescent endometriosis. J Adol Health Care 1:37, 1980.
6. Chatman D: Endometriosis in the black woman. Am J Obstet Gynecol 125:987, 1976.
7. Houston D: Evidence for the risk of pelvic endometriosis by age, race and economic status. Epidemiol Rev 6:167, 1984.
8. Schifrin B: Teen-age endometriosis. Am J Obstet Gynecol 116:973, 1973.
9. Sanfilippo J, Wakim N, Schikler K, Yussman M: Endometriosis in association with a uterine anomaly. Am J Obstet Gynecol 154:39, 1986.
10. Fallon J: Endometriosis in youth. JAMA 131:1405, 1946.
11. Derryberry W, Bonney W: Pelvic endometriosis in a 15 year old. Obstet Gynecol 27:558, 1968.
12. Bullock J, Massey F, Gambrell R: Symptomatic endometriosis in teenagers: a reappraisal. Obstet Gynecol 43:896, 1967.
13. Hanton E, Malkasian G, Dockerty M, et al.: Endometriosis in young women. Am J Obstet Gynecol 98:116, 1967.
14. Hanton E, Malkasian G, Dockerty M, et al.: Case report: endometriosis associated with complete or partial obstruction of menstrual egress. Obstet Gynecol 28:626, 1966.
15. Moore J, Schifrin B, Erez S: Ovarian tumors in infancy, childhood, and adolescence. Am J Obstet Gynecol 99:913, 1967.
16. Bruser N: The common occurrence of endometriosis in young women. Can Med Assoc J 72:190, 1955.
17. Depp O, Pope D: Early conservative surgery in endometriosis. South Med J 49:1345, 1956.
18. TeLinde R: Endometriosis. Clin Obstet Gynecol 4:788, 1961.
19. Sutton L: The clinical features of endometriosis. NY J Med 41:1343, 1941.
20. Sutton L: Etiologic factors in endometriosis with report of a case with reflux menstruation. NC Med J 31:45, 1970.
21. McDonald R: Uterus didelphys with endometriosis. Am J Obstet Gynecol 45:1038, 1943.
22. King W: Metastatic endometriosis and abdominal scars. Can J Surg 22:579, 1979.
23. Mittal G, Choudhury T, Cortez J: Endometriosis of the appendix presenting as acute appendicitis. Am J Surg 142:519, 1981.
24. Chatman D, Ward A: Endometriosis in adolescents. J Reprod Med 27:156, 1982.
25. Whitehouse H: Endometrioma invading the bladder removed from a patient who had never menstruated. Proc R Soc Med 19 (Obstet Gynecol Sec):15, 1925.
26. Seitz L: Uber genese, klinik und therapie der endometriosis (heterotopein der uterusschleimhaut). Arch Gynaekol 149:529, 1932.
27. Simpson J, Elias S, Malinak L, Buttram V: Heritable aspects of endometriosis. 1. Genetic studies. Am J Obstet Gynecol 137:327, 1980.
28. Bassler R, Theele Ch, Labach H: Nodular and tumorlike gliomatosis peritonei with endometriosis caused by a mature ovarian teratoma. Pathol Res Pract 175:392, 1982.
29. Pueblitz-Peredo S, Luevano-flores E, Rincon-Taracena R: Uteruslike mass of the ovary: endometriosis or congenital malformation. Arch Pathol Lab Med 109:361, 1985.
30. Acosta A, Kaplan A, Kaufman R: Gynecologic cancer in children. Am J Obstet Gynecol 112:944, 1972.
31. Bush W, Hall D, Ward B: Adenomyosis of the gastric antrum in children. Pediatr Radiol 111:179, 1974.

32. Huffman J: Endometriosis in young teen-age girls. Pediatr Ann 10:44, 1981.
33. Jones H: Reproductive impairment and the malformed uterus. Fertil Steril 36:137, 1981.
34. Barbieri R, Canick J, Makris A, Todd R, Davies I, Ryan K: Danazol inhibits steroidogenesis. Fertil Steril 28:809, 1977.
35. Luciano A, Hauser K, Chapler F, Wallace R: Effects of danazol on plasma lipid and lipoprotein levels in healthy women and in women with endometriosis. Am J Obstet Gynecol 145:422, 1983.
36. Betz G, Miller J, Hales D: Actions of danazol in vivo on cytochrome P-450 and steroidogenic enzymes in rat testis and liver microsomal preparations. Am J Obstet Gynecol 14:962, 1981.
37. Shaw R: Female pseudohermaphroditism associated with danazol exposure in utero case report. Br J Obstet Gynecol 91:386, 1984.
38. Thurell J, Dymling J: Effect of danazol on thryoid function in women. Postgrad Med J 55 (Suppl 5):33, 1979.
39. Buttram U Jr: Cyclic use of combination oral contraceptives and the severity of endometriosis. Fertil Steril 31:347, 1979.
40. Cramer D, Wilson E, Stillman R, Berger M, Belisle S, Schiff I, Albrecht B, Gibson M, Stadel B, Schoenbaum S: Association of endometriosis with oral contraceptive use. Presented at the American Fertility Society, Abstract 328, Toronto, 1986.
41. Ortiz A, Hiroi M, Stanczyk F, Goebelsman U, Mishell D: Serum medroxy-progesterone acetate (MPA) concentrations and ovarian function following intramuscular injection of Depo-MPA. J Clin Endocrinol Metab 44:32, 1977.

Endometriosis, pages 173–184

Chapter 10
Management of Recurrent Endometriosis

George M. Grunert, M.D., and Robert R. Franklin, M.D.

Department of Obstetrics and Gynecology, The Woman's Hospital of Texas, Baylor College of Medicine, Houston, Texas 77030

INTRODUCTION

In many respects, the literature serves as a poor guide for the clinician faced with the patient with recurrent endometriosis following conservative therapy. Reports of incidence, guidelines for management, and results of therapy for patients with recurrent endometriosis are sparse. Discussions of radical surgery for endometriosis generally involve only the mention of hysterectomy for benign disease, without specific consideration for the nature of endometriosis.

In this chapter we discuss pitfalls encountered in initial conservative surgery and attempt to formulate a rational plan of management based both on written reports and on extensive personal experience for the patient with recurrent disease. Specifically, we examine preoperative evaluation and preparation, specifics of surgical technique, results of surgery, and subsequent management. In addition, we discuss radical surgery for endometriosis, i.e., surgery involving hysterectomy with or without adnexectomy, and the approach to the patient with recurrence after radical surgery.

PREOPERATIVE CONSIDERATIONS

Pitfalls at Initial Surgery

Current information suggests that visible endometriosis is frequently accompanied by microscopic peritoneal involvement [1]. It should not be surprising that persistent or recurrent endometriosis is common. It now appears that conservative resection of endometriosis should be placed in the category of cytoreductive rather than curative surgery. While previous series have documented recurrence of symptoms attributed to endometriosis, the observed incidence of recurrence is now increased by the use of laparoscopy for the evaluation of continuing infertility without other symptoms.

The most common error made at initial surgery is incomplete resection of gross disease. While microscopic disease cannot be excised, an aggressive approach to conservative surgery must be maintained. Inadequate preoperative evaluation or preparation, an injudiciously timid approach to surgery, a lack of appreciation for the natural history of the disease, and the feeling that medical therapy will somehow take care of lesions that are difficult to remove, may all contribute to recurrence. The failure to completely resect cul-de-sac or rectosigmoid implants is common. Residual ovarian disease may be left because of a failure to appreciate the convoluted nature of endometriomas or because of a reluctance to approach an ovary adherent over the ureter. We discuss specific approaches to these areas below.

Because it is difficult to differentiate symptoms of endometriosis from those of adhesions subsequent to surgery, surgery may be indicated in the absence of anatomic recurrence. The use of careful surgical technique, attention to hemostasis and reperitonealization of raw surfaces, and the use of adjuvant agents to decrease adhesions at initial surgery all contribute to decreased adhesion formation. If extensive peritoneal defects are left, the adnexae may adhere into the cul-de-sac, compromising fertility and producing pain. Accordionlike adhesions of the rectosigmoid result from mobilization of the sigmoid without reconstruction of its support and may lead to postoperative bowel symptoms in the absence of active endometriosis.

In patients who have undergone hysterectomy and adnexectomy, recurrence is most commonly associated with residual functional ovarian tissue. This is usually a result of incomplete resection of the ovary by including ovarian tissue in the initial ovarian pedicle clamp. This can be avoided by ligating the ovarian vascular supply high on the pelvic sidewall with the ureter in view. The ovary is then carefully dissected away from the sidewall and can be completely removed. In rare cases, an accessory ovary is noted on the sidewall. A careful inspection should be made to rule out this possibility.

Preoperative Evaluation

Recurrence must be considered in the light of previous treatment, present symptoms, and future reproductive desires of the patient. For purposes of discussion, we will divide patients into three groups: those who have had conservative therapy and desire fertility, those who no longer desire fertility, and those who have recurrence following radical surgery.

Documentation and appropriate staging of recurrent endometriosis is critical, both for diagnosis and treatment planning. Symptoms may be due to adhesions or other pelvic abnormalities in the absence of active endometriosis. The appearance of adnexal masses or cul-de-sac nodularity in a patient previously treated for endometriosis may represent diseases other than endometriosis. An inappropriate conclusion that pelvic abnormalities are due to endometriosis may lead to erroneous therapy and may potentially delay appropriate treatment of a pelvic neoplasm.

Recurrence rates following conservative therapy are difficult to estimate accurately, with rates from 2% to 47% having been quoted [2–6]. The incidence is largely dependent on length of follow-up and diligence of evaluation. Wheeler and Malinak, in a retrospective study of patients following conservative surgery, found a cumulative recurrence rate of 13.5% at 3 years and 40.3% at 5 years [7]. There was no significant difference based on initial staging or conception following initial surgery. These data differed from other studies in that patients without symptoms underwent laparoscopy if pregnancy did not follow the initial surgery.

Recurrent symptoms following pseudopregnancy regimens vary from 17% to 29% [4,8,9]. Following danazol therapy alone, symptoms were reported in 38% of patients by Puleo and Hammond [10] and in 33% by Greenblatt and Tzingounis [11]. Asymptomatic patients with recurrence were not noted in these studies, so the true recurrence rate may have been higher.

In patients desirous of fertility, it is difficult to give an exact plan for management because of the sparsity of data in the literature. Prior to concluding that the endometriosis is the direct cause of infertility, a thorough, contemporary review of the general infertility evaluation must be done. As found by Schenken and Malinak, the coexistence of a male factor, an anatomic tubal factor, or multiple factors severely decreases the expected success of surgery [12]. An effort must be made to identify and treat all other factors prior to proceeding to surgery. There is little information regarding medical therapy following initial treatment. It may merit consideration in patients without significant anatomic distortion of the pelvis.

Recurrence following radical surgery is less common. Ranney [13] reported symptomatic recurrence in 3% of patients treated by total abdominal hysterectomy and bilateral salpingo-oophorectomy who were given estrogen replacement. He similarly found only a 0.7% recurrence rate when there was ovarian preservation at the initial radical surgery [14]. Documentation of the diagnosis is essential to proper therapy; however, the risk of laparoscopy in these patients must be weighed against the possible risk of a delayed diagnosis.

Patients with endogenous ovarian activity may be candidates for medical therapy, be it with progestins, danazol, or GnRH analogs. The expected response to therapy must be individualized based on extent and location of disease as well as previous response to therapy. While an initial trial of medical therapy is not unreasonable in some patients, poor response to therapy or progression of physical findings mandates exploration. The patient with significant anatomic distortion due to adhesions, with ovarian endometriomas, or who previously failed to respond to medical therapy, is a better candidate for surgery than for medical suppression.

Recurrence following hysterectomy with bilateral salpingo-oophorectomy should make one suspicious of the presence of residual functional ovarian tissue in these patients. Estrogen and progestin replacement is only rarely associated with regrowth of endometriosis. The initial approach is to discontinue hormonal replacement and measure gonadotropins. If FSH levels are not in the menopausal range, recurrence is most likely associated with persistent ovarian function. Uncertain results can be evaluated using an hCG stimulation test: a baseline entradiol and testosterone are drawn, followed by the administration of 10,000 units of hCG. A doubling of baseline values at 48 hours is consistent with ovarian function.

Although medical therapy in the absence of ovarian function carries a low chance of response, there may be individual patients who benefit by the reduction of estrogen receptors within the endometriosis itself. This presumes that there is sufficient peripheral production of estrogen to stimulate growth. Progestins, androgens, danazol, or antiestrogens may be helpful in selected cases.

Because many of these patients come to surgery for pain, they frequently have been using analgesics such as aspirin and the nonsteroidal antiinflammatory drugs. These may prolong the bleeding time and should, therefore, be avoided preoperatively. Oral contraceptives, once advocated preoperatively, may increase the risk of thrombophlebitis. We frequently utilize preoperative treatment with danazol, using a 3-month course of 800 mg per day, feeling that this decreases endometriotic vascularity and, combined with surgery, appears to improve postoperative pregnancy rates.

A history of previous ovarian surgery, adnexal masses or immobility, or GU symptoms are indications for a preoperative intravenous pyelogram (IVP). This serves as a rough guide to ureteral position but more importantly alerts one to the possibility of ureteral duplication. It also may identify the occasional patient with preoperative ureteral obstruction, which might not otherwise be noted until after surgery. Hematuria is an indication for cystoscopy in addition to IVP. If the gynecologist is not specifically trained in the management of ureteral and bladder involvement, a urologist should be utilized as an intraoperative consultant.

In a similar fashion, patients with GI symptoms, rectal fixation, nodularity of the rectovaginal septum, cul-de-sac obliteration, or extensive endometriosis should have a barium enema and sigmoidoscopy prior to laparotomy. Other GI testing should be performed as indicated. If there is any question of bowel involvement, we utilize a preoperative mechanical and antibiotic bowel prep. It is always preferable to prep a patient who does not require bowel surgery than to run the risk of not prepping a patient who does. As above, if one anticipates the need for assistance in bowel surgery, a general or colon-rectal surgeon should be involved in the surgery.

It must be appreciated that the patient who has undergone extensive evaluation and treatment for infertility, usually involving multiple operative procedures, who elects hysterectomy for relief of symptoms, is making a tremendously important decision. She should be given the opportunity to discuss her feelings freely and should be offered professional counseling and referral to support groups as appropriate. The possibility of oophorectomy and postoperative hormonal replacement should be clearly outlined.

SURGICAL TECHNIQUE

The Patient Who Desires Fertility

We favor the judicious use of operative and laser laparoscopy where feasible. Each second-look laparoscopy is planned as a possible laser laparoscopy, using the laparoscopically directed carbon dioxide laser. Patients with accessible mild or moderate disease or with relatively avascular adhesions without gross anatomic distortion are candidates for laser laparoscopy. Specific techniques are described elsewhere in this text.

If laparotomy is indicated, one must be prepared to deal not only with the endometriosis itself but with adhesions due to the previous operative procedure. Adequate visualization is mandatory, especially with exposure of the lateral pelvis and cul-de-sac. We have found the transverse incision to be ideal for exposure and for its strength and healing characteristics. If lateral exposure must be increased, the recti may be transected, although this is rarely necessary. In cases where access to the upper abdomen is necessary, a transverse skin incision can be made, the abdominal wall dissected from the fascia, and a vertical fascial incision made.

Upon entering the abdomen, careful attention must be paid to the possibility of adhesions to previous surgical sites. The combined effect of endometriosis and multiple surgeries may frequently distort pelvic anatomy. The first aim should be to restore normal anatomic relationships and to identify all structures. It is generally best to begin working from the lateral pelvis medially, and then from above downward once lateral mobilization has been achieved.

Meticulous atraumatic microsurgical technique with specific attention to hemostasis is used. The aim is to resect or remove all visible disease and restore anatomic normality. This may include any and all aspects of pelvic reconstructive surgery in addition to the excision or vaporization of endometriosis. Pelvic adhesions are excised, not divided. Peritoneal defects are carefully closed to decrease the possibility of adhesions. We utilize the microscopically controlled carbon dioxide laser for these procedures. The laser facilitates excision of endometriomas and, combined with preoperative danazol, reduces the need for wedge resection or oophorectomy. While unilateral severe endometriosis is best approached with salpingo-oophorectomy, we attempt to preserve ovarian tissue if possible. Should the surgery itself fail to result in pregnancy, this may improve the chances of oocyte retrieval for in-vitro fertilization.

Presacral neurectomy, if not performed at the first laparotomy, is recommended. Uterine suspension, utilizing the round ligaments, may be indicated to elevate the adnexae out of the cul-de-sac during the healing phase. Plication of the uterosacral ligaments may be necessary following resection and may assist in reperitonealization. Danazol is continued postoperatively for 1 month in patients with resection of ovarian disease to prevent immediate ovulation, which might disrupt suture lines. Hyskon (32% Dextran 70 in dextrose) is instilled into the pelvis at the terminaton of surgery to reduce the incidence of postoperative adhesions.

The Patient Who No Longer Desires Fertility

The patient who no longer desires fertility may also be managed by laparoscopic surgery if feasible. If not, she may be offered symptomatic relief, medical therapy, or conservative surgery, but she is a more appropriate candidate for radical surgery. Radical surgery for endometriosis is defined as that surgery that removes the uterus, with or without adnexae. Hysterectomy for endometriosis may be a simple procedure for benign disease or may be as difficult as radical pelvic surgery.

We will not address the technique of abdominal hysterectomy per se, except to note specific variations of technique related to endometriosis. Although intrafascial hysterectomy is taught as a safeguard against ureteral injury, we prefer an extrafascial technique after the ureters have been identified. This reduces the possibility of leaving residual endometriosis.

The question of when to perform oophorectomy at the time of definitive surgery for endometriosis is difficult to answer. Most studies indicate that preservation of a normal ovary is associated with a 5–10% chance of postoperative recurrence [14–16]. It is our practice to leave an uninvolved ovary except in cases of extensive endometriosis. If endometriosis cannot be completely excised or if there is extensive bilateral ovarian involvement, the preferred technique is en bloc removal of the uterus and adnexae to minimize leaving residual disease. In selected cases, it may be advantageous to separate the adnexae from the uterus first, perform the hysterectomy, and then perform the adnexectomy.

In making a posterior peritoneal incision for hysterectomy, care should be taken to ensure that endometriosis implants are excised. If there is uterosacral ligament involvement, it is best to identify and ligate the peritoneal reflection of the ligaments away from the uterus, including cul-de-sac endometriosis with the hysterectomy specimen (Fig. 1). Lateral pelvic sidewall peritoneum

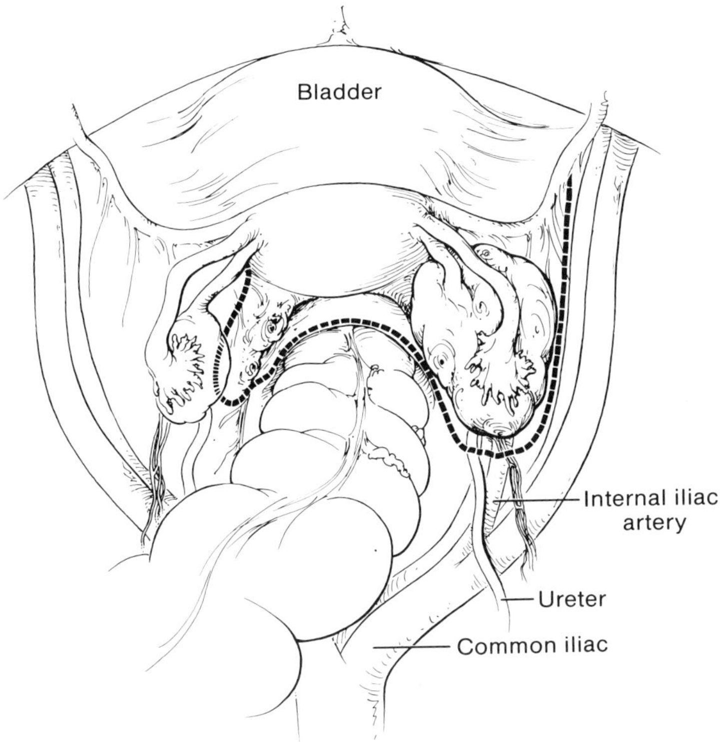

Fig. 1. Placement of the posterior peritoneal incision must be individualized. On the left, the uterosacral reflection is excised away from the uterus to remove endometriosis. On the right, pelvic sidewall peritoneum is included for en-bloc removal.

should also be excised if involved. Because this may approach the ureter, it should be visualized in its entire course prior to uterosacral resection.

Genitourinary tract. Intraoperative ureteral identification is mandatory. While some favor the preoperative placement of ureteral catheters, we have not found this technique especially useful, and have seen ureteral transection despite catheterization. If the broad ligament is free, the ureter may be identified in the base of the ligament either following transection of the round ligament (Fig. 2) or by opening the peritoneum between the broad and infundibulopelvic ligaments. Because the ovary may be densely adherent to the ovarian fossa over the ureter, an alternative approach to the ureter is to identify it as it crosses over the pelvic brim (Fig. 3). It may then be traced through the pelvis as the ovarian and uterine vessels are ligated with the ureter in view.

In cases where a uterosacral resection has been performed at previous conservative surgery, the ureter may be drawn away from the sidewall toward the midline. Again, careful identification and protection are mandatory.

Superficial endometriosis overlying the ureter may be excised or laser vaporized. To protect the ureter from inadvertent laser injury, it may be useful to inject saline under peritoneal implants so that the beam is absorbed by the water after the implant has been vaporized. More extensive ureteral involvement may require local resection and anastomosis or reimplantation. Where this is anticipated preoperatively, it is far better to be prepared to involve a urologist than to run the risk of an incomplete operation.

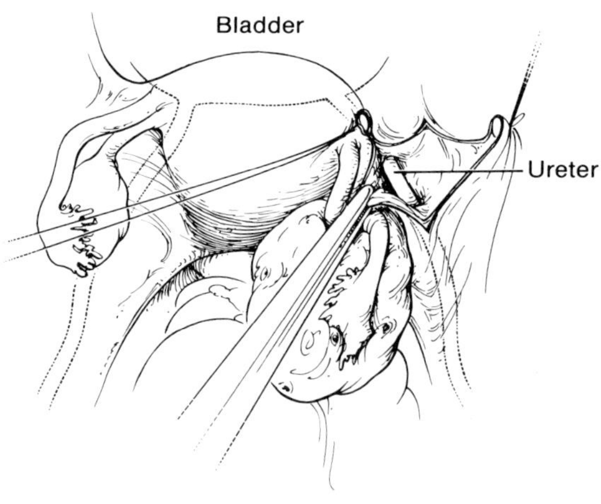

Fig. 2. The ureter can be located on the medial leaf of the broad ligament beneath the transected round ligament.

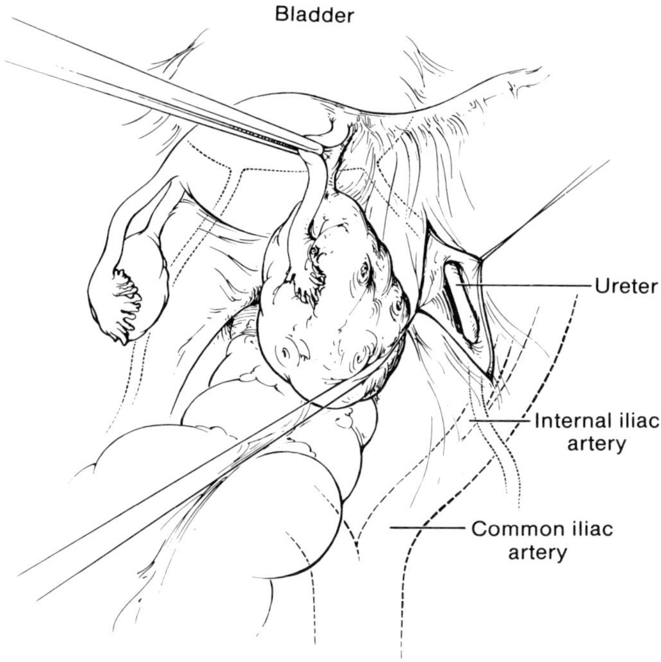

Fig. 3. The ureter can be identified as it crosses over the pelvic brim and passes over and medial to the internal iliac artery.

Bladder involvement may be approached by local excision or vaporization of superficial implants. Invasive disease requires incision into and occasionally through the wall of the bladder for removal. If there is any question of deep involvement, the dome of the bladder should be opened so that the excision can be carried out with the trigone and ureteral orifices in view.

Gastrointestinal tract. Long-term experience in dealing with patients with bowel endometriosis has led us to an increasingly aggressive approach to these lesions [17]. Superficial lesions may be treated by fulguration, laser vaporization, or observation. Locally invasive lesions are best treated by local excision or wedge resection with layered closure. The intestinal wall should be closed transversely to decrease the possibility of postoperative stenosis.

Lesions that are transmural, that involve more than one-half the circumference of the bowel, or that involve more length than can be removed with a wedge resection should be treated with segmental resection. In the properly prepared patient, primary reanastomosis is performed. It is advantageous to place the anastomosis line below the posterior peritoneal reflection. If this is not possible, the uterosacral ligaments can be plicated over the suture line so that the adnexae do not adhere to the site.

POSTOPERATIVE CONSIDERATIONS

Results of second conservative operations, defined as pregnancy rates, have been difficult to determine. Schenken and Malinak [17] reported a 12% pregnancy rate. Wheeler and Malinak [7], however, in a subsequent report including the same patients, noted a 47% pregnancy rate within 18 months of surgery if recurrent endometriosis was found, and a 60% pregnancy rate if no active disease was noted. In this series, 20% of patients required a third laparotomy.

Adding to the dilemma of therapy in this group is the ongoing development of Gamete Intrafallopian Transfer (GIFT) and In-vitro Fertilization (IVF) programs. Ultimately, the success of these techniques, combined with results of embryo cryopreservation, will have to be compared with results of secondary therapy. It appears that GIFT or IVF may be the preferred route of management in the patient with recurrent mild or moderate endometriosis who desires pregnancy. The exception is that patient who requires therapy directed at the endometriosis itself for symptomatic relief.

In the patient who is actively trying for pregnancy, the concurrent evaluation and treatment of other factors must be continued. We recommend a second-look laparoscopy at 6 to 12 months to both treat adhesions and recurrent endometriosis and to serve as a prognostic guide. It may be appropriate to include GIFT with this laparoscopy as an additional therapeutic modality. Based on laparoscopic findings, an appropriate therapeutic direction may be chosen.

Third attempts at conservative surgery have generally been unsatisfactory and should be discouraged. Although there may be that individual patient with extenuating circumstances or a completely new facet to her disease, results have been uniformly poor.

Postoperative hormonal replacement following radical surgery remains controversial. The slight risk of stimulation of disease must be weighed against the need for symptomatic relief and prophylaxis of osteoporosis. We feel the advantages far outweigh the rare disadvantages and recommend replacement in a physiologic fashion with continuous lowdose estrogen replacement and cyclic progestin replacement. Supplemental calcium and exercise programs must also be emphasized. Patients with symptomatic recurrence on replacement estrogens and progestins who do not have evidence of endogenous ovarian function can usually be managed by temporary discontinuation of therapy until symptoms subside.

COMMENT

Endometriosis is a disease that is rarely fatal to the patient. It may, however, prevent conception and be as symptomatically devastating as any fatal illness. For the most part, it is a disease of coping: coping with discomfort, dyspareunia, dysmenorrhea, marital disruptions, infertility, frequent trips to physicians and hospitals, multiple regimens of medical therapy, multiple operations, and extreme frustration. The careful physician, by meticulously documenting the disease and applying the principles of medical and surgical therapies, can often offer an improvement in fertility chances and a decrease in symptoms. It is important to avoid the tendency to treat without a definitive diagnosis or plan of action. Proper treatment may involve multiple modalities and multiple specialties and can humble even the most skilled surgeon. Above all, the patient must be accurately informed about her disease and treatment alternatives so she can be intimately involved in all decisions made regarding care.

REFERENCES

1. Murphy AA, Green WR, Bobbie D, dela Cruz ZC, Rock JA: Unsuspected endometriosis documented by scanning electron microscopy in visually normal peritoneum. Fertil Steril 46:522, 1986.
2. Green RH Jr: Conservative surgical treatment of endometriosis. Clin Obstet Gynecol 9:293, 1966.
3. Andrews WC, Larsen GD: Endometriosis: treatment with hormonal pseudopregnancy and/or operation. Am J Obstet Gynecol 118:643, 1974.
4. Andrews WC: Medical versus surgical treatment of endometriosis. Clin Obstet Gynecol 23:917, 1980.
5. Punnonnen R, Klemi P, Nikkanen V: Recurrent endometriosis. Gynecol Obstet Invest 11:307, 1980.
6. Gordts S, Boecks W, Brosens I: Microsurgery of endometriosis in infertile patients. Fertil Steril 42:520, 1984.
7. Wheeler JM, Malinak LR: Recurrent endometriosis: incidence, management, and prognosis. Am J Obstet Gynecol 146:247, 1983.
8. Riva HL, Wilson JH, Kawaskai DM: Effect of norethynodrel on endometriosis. Am J Obstet Gynecol 82:109, 1961.
9. Kistner RW: Infertility with endometriosis. A plan of therapy. Fertil Steril 13:237, 1962.
10. Puleo JG, Hammond CB: Conservative treatment of endometriosis externa: the effects of danazol therapy. Fertil Steril 40:164, 1983.
11. Greenblatt RB, Tzingounis V: Danazol treatment of endometriosis: long-term follow-up. Fertil Steril 32:518, 1979.

12. Schenken RS, Malinak LR: Reoperation after initial treatment of endometriosis with conservative surgery. Am J Obstet Gynecol 131:416, 1978.
13. Ranney B: Endometriosis. III. Complete operations. Am J Obstet Gynecol 109:1137, 1971.
14. Ranney B: Endometriosis. I. Conservative operations. Am J Obstet Gynecol 107:743, 1970.
15. Counseler VS, Crenshaw JL Jr.: A clinical and surgical review of endometriosis. Am J Obstet Gynecol 62:930, 1951.
16. Andrews SC, Larsen GD: Endometriosis: treatment with hormonal pseudopregnancy and/or operation. Am J Obstet Gynecol 121:283, 1975.
17. Williams TJ, Pratt JH: Endometriosis in 1000 consecutive celiotomies: incidence and management. Am J Obstet Gynecol 129:245, 1977.
18. Wheeler JM, Maxey T, Christy RK, Young RL, Franklin RR, Buttram VB, Malinak LR: Gastrointestinal endometriosis: Evaluation of four treatment options at conservative laparotomy for pelvic endometriosis. Presented at the Forty-first Annual Meeting of the American Fertility Society, September 30, 1985.

Endometriosis, pages 185–206

Chapter 11
Extra Pelvic Endometriosis

John A. Rock, M.D., and Sanford M. Markham, M.D.

Department of Gynecology and Obstetrics, Division of Reproductive Endocrinology, The Johns Hopkins Hospital, Baltimore, Maryland 21205

INTRODUCTION

Since the first report of endometriosis by Rokitansky in 1860 [1], interest in extra pelvic or nongynecologic endometriosis has had a special fascination because of the diversity of reported sites of ectopic endometrium and the unusual symptoms and complaints frequently present with this entity. In addition to endometriosis of the uterus, tubes, ovaries, and peritoneum covering these structures, medical textbooks and journals have documented ectopic sites such as the appendix [2], the bladder [3], the cervix [4], extremities [5], hernia sacs [6], inguinal region [7], nerves [8], the pleural cavity and lungs [9], rectum [10], round ligaments [1], lymph glands [11], sigmoid colon [12], small intestine [13], umbilicus [14], vagina [6], and the vulva [15] (Figs. 1, 2). The symptoms and complaints associated with extra pelvic endometriosis are quite diverse and usually relate to the physiologic function of the ectopic site. Though symptomatology in extra pelvic endometriosis is usually related to the menstrual cycle, in some patients this has not occurred, making the diagnosis confusing. Treatment has been most successful with either hormonal suppression or surgical removal. Ovarian ablation usually cures the disease.

ETIOLOGY OF EXTRA PELVIC ENDOMETRIOSIS

The etiology of endometriosis has most commonly been attributed to either the transport theory or the coelomic metaplasia theory [15]. The transport

Sanford M. Markham is an AFIT Fellow at the Wright-Patterson Air Force Base, Ohio.

The opinions expressed herein are those of the authors and not necessarily those of the United States Air Force or the Department of Defense.

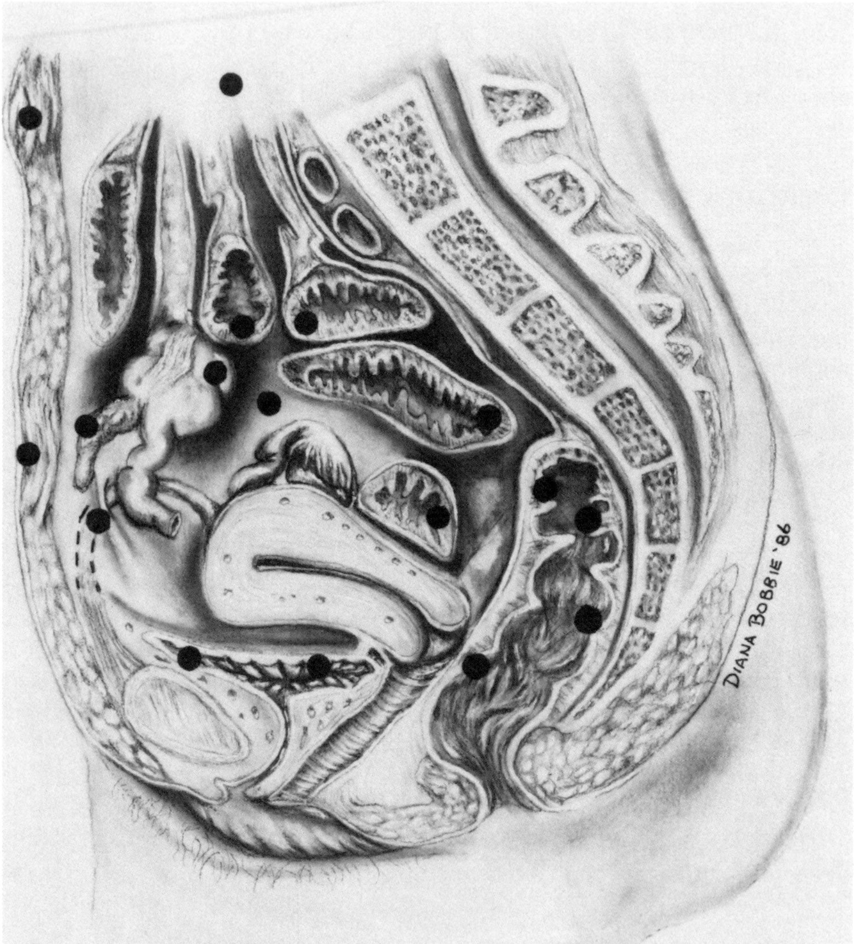

Fig. 1. Common sites of endometriosis in the pelvis.

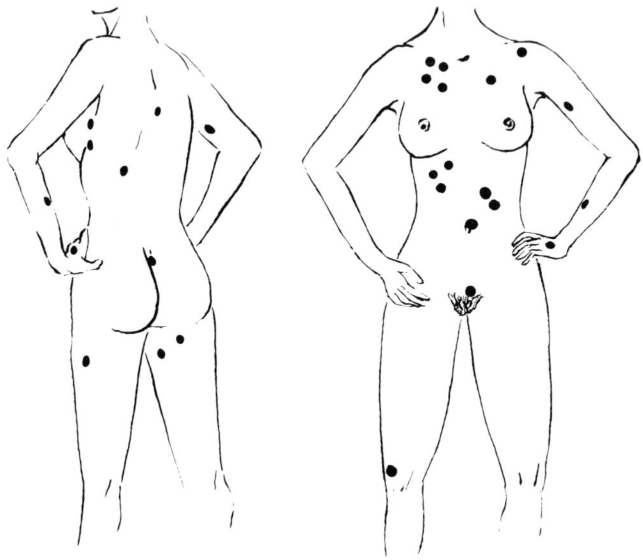

Fig. 2. Endometriosis reported at extra pelvic sites.

theory includes both retrograde regurgitation of endometrium through the oviducts and/or transport of endometrium via vascular channels or lymphatics to distant sites. This theory would seem to be the most likely in consideration of extra pelvic endometriosis, particularly with endometriosis found outside of the abdominal cavity. A mechanical transplant etiology has been thought to be most likely in endometriosis appearing in old abdominal and perineal incision sites. The coelomic metaplasia theory, which implies a metaplasia of pelvic and abdominal peritoneum into mullerian elements, such as endometrium, cannot be discounted. Since either theory fails to fully explain the vastly divergent sites of ectopic endometriosis, it is possible that a combination of the transport and metaplasia theories can be used to explain the occurrence of extra pelvic endometriosis. The incidence of endometriosis has been reported as high as 36% by Meigs [17] (1949) to 5–15% by Barbieri and Kistner [16] (1986). It is the impression of Williams [18] that the incidence of extra pelvic endometriosis decreases as the centrifugal distance from the uterus increases. A review of literature since 1980 would tend to support this impression, with the higher incidence of extra genital sites of endometriosis occurring in the large and small bowel, appendix, and urinary tract (Table I).

TABLE I. Incidence of Extra Pelvic Endometriosis

A. Incidence of endometriosis		
Kistner, 1986 [16]	5%–15% of women between 25 and 35 years of age undergoing laparotomy	
Ranney, 1980 [28]	4%–17% of menstruating women	
Meyers, 1979 [29]	8%–15%	
Williams and Pratt, 1977 [25]	38%	
Meigs, 1941 [30]	36% of 400 consecutive patients at laparotomy	
B. Incidence of extra pelvic endometriosis		
Kistner, 1986 [16]	Small bowel	0.1%–0.2%
Williams, 1985 [18]	Omentum	0.6%
	Small intestine	0.2%
	Appendix	1.4%
	Sigmoid colon	0.8%
	Inguinal	0.8%
	Umbilical	0.8%
	Incisional, ventral	0.8%
	Incisional, vulva	0.2%
Gitelis, 1985 [31]	Lung and pleura	51.0% (of extra abdominal endometriosis)
Yates-Bell, 1972 [19]	Urinary tract	1.0%
Ball and Platt, 1962 [20]	Urinary tract	0.5%
Macafee and Greer, 1960 [23]	Intestine	12.0%
Lane, 1960 [2]	Appendix	<1.0%
Scott, 1950 [32]	Appendix	1.4%

In a large series of patients with abdominal endometriosis reviewed by Williams [18], the incidence of extra genital endometriosis was as follows: omentum, 0.6%; small intestine, 0.2%; appendix, 1.4%; sigmoid, 0.8%; inguinal canal, 0.8%; umbilicus, 0.8%; incision, ventral, 0.8%; incision, vulval, 0.2%. He additionally reported a 2.5% incidence of endometriosis of the cervix. Barbieri and Kistner [16] have reported an incidence of 0.1–0.2% of endometriosis of small bowel, and Yates-Bell et al. [18] and Ball and Platt [20] have reported an incidence of endometriosis of the urinary tract between 0.5% and 1.0%. These numbers would tend to indicate a low incidence of extra pelvic endometriosis. They would also suggest that this diagnosis should always be considered in lesions outside of the pelvis, particularly with cyclic manifestations.

PATHOLOGY AND HISTOLOGY

A key factor in the pathogenesis of extra pelvic endometriosis is the hormonal relationship. Like pelvic endometriosis, it is uncommon prior to menarche and after menopause. Novak [6], however, has recorded an endometrioma appearing in a McBurney scar in a patient whose appendectomy was done prior to menarche. Ovarian suppression or ablation commonly results in prompt and complete regression of symptoms of extra pelvic endometriosis. Excision of implants of extra pelvic endometriosis may reveal endometrial epithelium, glandlike structures, and/or stroma with hemorrhage. Continued cyclic stimulation of areas of ectopic endometriosis results in eventual obliteration of its microscopic pattern, and thus it has been reported by Hertig that "The more advanced the lesion clinically, the poorer the histologic detail" [16].

Extra pelvic endometriosis has been reported in a variety of histologic patterns varying from typical endometrial glands to an abundance of fibrostroma. Cystic variations have been more common in pulmonary endometriosis and a combination of glandular and stromal growth in lesions involving the intestinal tract. In either case, it is common to observe cyclic changes not unlike those found in endometrium in the uterus. Pregnancy or pseudopregnancy frequently results in decidual reaction similar to that seen in pelvic endometriosis. Of significance is the fact that the histologic pattern of extra pelvic endometriosis may only exhibit proliferative changes without a secretory pattern.

CLINICAL CHARACTERISTICS AND FEATURES

The location of extra pelvic or nongynecological endometriosis can best be divided into four anatomic regions: 1) pulmonary endometriosis, 2) bowel-omental endometriosis, 3) urinary tract endometriosis, and 4) endometriosis of other sites. Though pelvic endometriosis has been carefully classified by the American Fertility Society into stages depending upon the degree and extent of involvement, extra pelvic endometriosis lacks that approach because of the vastly different sites of involvement and the diversity of symptoms.

Pulmonary Endometriosis

The signs and symptoms of pulmonary endometriosis include usually hemothorax, pneumothorax, or hemoptysis concurrent with menses. Karpel et al. [21] recently reported a review of 84 cases of pulmonary endometriosis, which included 63 cases with catamenial pneumothorax, 9 cases of catamenial hemothorax, and 7 cases of catamenial hemoptysis. Of the patients with hemothorax, all had extensive pelvic endometriosis. However, the patients with hemoptysis had no evidence of pelvic endometriosis. Foster et al. [9] have reviewed 65 cases of pulmonary endometriosis, which were subdivided into pleural and parenchymal disease. The authors noted that women with pleural endometriosis were younger than those with parenchymal disease, and patients with pleural disease presented with pain and dyspnea associated with right-sided pneumothorax or pleural effusion in 93% of the cases. There appeared to be no difference in parity between the two categories. Prior pelvic surgery for other complaints was significantly more common in the parenchymal group compared with the pleural group.

The etiology of pulmonary endometriosis is most likely through a transport mechanism either involving direct spread of endometrial implants to the pleural cavity by way of diaphragmatic defects or through lymphatic vessels or vascular channels. Of the cases reported by Karpel [21] with catamenial pneumothorax, 33% were found to have perforations of the diaphragm. An additional 35% were noted to have endometrial implants on the diaphragm and/or the pleura. It would seem likely therefore that thoracic cavity endometriosis occurs as a result of direct spread of pelvic endometriosis through the diaphragm. However, the possibility of lymphatic or vascular transmission cannot be ruled out. In those with hemothorax, all had extensive pelvic endometriosis, while in those with pneumothorax just under one-quarter had pelvic endometriosis and, in those with hemoptysis, none had evidence of pelvic endometriosis. Of the patients with pneumothorax who underwent thoracotomy and/or biopsy, only 35% were found to have endometrial implants and a definitive diagnosis established. In 25% of the cases, no abnormal findings were discovered. In the patients with hemothorax, thoracotomy was performed in seven of the nine cases and thoracic pleural endometriosis was found in five. Of the patients with catamenial hemoptysis, bleeding was localized by rigid bronchoscopy or thoracotomy. Endometrial tissue was found in all who underwent thoracotomy. In the cases presented by Foster et al. [9], 41 of the 54 cases underwent thoracotomy and in 80% of these, endometriosis was diagnosed by biopsy. Implants of endometriosis were described or a biopsy revealed fibrosis and hemosiderin depositions in the remaining 13 women. Of the two series reported by Foster et al. [19] and Karpel et al. [21], there was a predominance of right-sided lesions in 93% and 95% of the women respectively. A review of individual patients published since 1980 would tend to support the predominance of right-sided pulmonary endometriosis (Table II).

Successful therapy in these reported cases would tend to favor operative intervention with thoracotomy and pleurodesis either by chemical or abrasive means in more advanced cases. In some cases, however, total abdominal hysterectomy and salpingo-oophorectomy became necessary to control symptoms of pulmonary endometriosis and/or progressive pelvic endometriosis. The use of chemical suppression by means of danazol, medroxyprogesterone, or birth control pills, etc., has in most cases provided some temporary relief. The most effective therapy in pulmonary endometriosis is bronchoscopy and/or thoracentesis followed by thoracotomy with excision of endometriotic lesions, pleurodesis, and repair of diaphragmatic perforations when found.

Our therapeutic recommendations are based on the patient's age and fertility status. Conservative therapy (i.e., hormonal therapy) may be in order if the patient wishes to maintain her reproductive capacity. Thoracotomy should only be considered when there is a discrete lesion or if recurrent pneumothorax requires pleural abrasion. If fertility is not an issue, then oophorectomy, with or without hysterectomy, is indicated for relief of symptoms. Interestingly, symptoms do not usually recur with low-dose estrogen replacement. The use of radiation either directly to endometriosis of the lung or pleura or as a form of castration would appear to have no advantage over surgery or hormonal suppression.

Intestinal Endometriosis

Endometriosis of the intestinal tract, including small bowel, large bowel, and omentum, represents the most common site for endometriosis outside of the uterus, fallopian tubes, ovaries, and peritoneum surrounding these structures. Forsgren [22] has reported colon and rectal endometriosis in 17 of 139 patients (12%) who were treated for symptomatic endometriosis. Of this number, 6 were referred for surgery having symptoms compatible with bowel obstruction. Surgical intervention was dependent upon the extent of the lesion found and varied from resection to release of sigmoidal obstruction. Macafee and Greer [23] reviewed several series of endometriosis totaling over 7,000 patients and found intestinal involvement in 12%. Of these, 72.4% had involvement of the sigmoid colon and/or rectum. In a review of intestinal endometriosis reported since 1980, involvement of the colon occurred in 25 of the 35 patients reported (Table III).

Treatment of rectal or colonic endometriosis has varied depending upon the extent of disease and the location of involvement. Our therapeutic recommendations would favor the use of hormone suppression such as estrogen-progesterone combinations in the form of birth control pills, medroxyprogesterone, and/or danazol. In severe cases of endometriosis or following failure of hormonal management, conservative or definitive surgical intervention is required. Conservative procedures would include excisional biopsy as well as local excision with or without dilatation of the involved bowel segment. Definitive procedures would include segmental resection of the bowel or anterior resection with total abdominal hysterectomy and bilateral salpingo-oophorectomy (Fig. 3). Colon surgery should not be attempted without a preoperative mechanical and nonabsorbable antibiotic bowel preparation.

TABLE II. Clinical Data - Pulmonary Endometriosis and Catamenial Events

Author	Age	Pulmonary symptoms	Gynecologic symptoms	Previous OB/GYN surgery	Operative procedure	Diagnosis
Suginami, 1985 [33]	25	Hemoptysis, severe cough	Symptoms worse with menses, irregular cycles	Elective abortion	Laparoscopy, bronchoscopy with biopsy (danazol), resection of upper lobe of right lung	Endometriosis of the pelvis and upper lobe of the right lung
Karpel, 1985 [21]	25	Right-sided pleuritic	Symptoms concurrent with menses	Unknown	Chemical pleurodesis thoracotomy with closure of diaphragmatic perforations and abrasive pleurodesis	Catamenial pneumothorax
	42	Dyspnea and right shoulder pain, pleural effusion	Symptoms concurrent with menses	Unknown	Thoracentesis, (danazol), chemical pleurodesis, thoracotomy, excision of hemorrhagic cyst, pleural decortication	Catamenial hemothorax
	31	Hemoptysis, pleuritic chest pain	Symptoms concurrent with menses	Unknown	Bronchoscopy with biopsy (followed by planned pregnancies)	Catamenial hemoptysis
Wilkins, 1985 [34]	32	Dyspnea, cough, increasing abdominal girth, pleural effusion	Symptoms not related to menses, menses shorter since onset of symptoms	Unknown	Thoracentesis, tube thoracotomy, pleural biopsy	Pleural endometriosis with recurrent hemothorax, pelvic endometriosis, severe
Foster, 1981 [9]	30	Right-sided chest pain, right pneumothorax	Symptoms associated with menses, infertility	Unknown	Thoracentesis, (danazol), thoractomy, apical pleurectomy, excision of endometrial nodules	Pleural endometriosis
	24	Dyspnea, opacification of the right lung field	Lower abdominal pain and a pelvic mass	Unknown	Thoracentesis, (danazol), pleurectomy, excision of endometrial implants and oversewing of diaphragmatic defects	Pleural endometriosis, Pelvic endometriosis

	36	Recurrent hemoptysis	Symptoms associated with menses	Previous cesarean	Bronchoscopy, bronchial washings, (danazol)	Pulmonary endometriosis
Hibbard, 1981 [35]	48	Intermittent right upper chest pain, chronic bronchitis, bronchiectasis, right emphysema with surgical drainage (past history)	Symptoms associated with menses	Unknown	(Depo-Provera, Premarin) TAH, BSO	Catamenial pneumothorax, Pelvic endometriosis, severe
	28	Hemorrhagic pleural effusion	(Implied cyclic symptoms)	Unknown	Thoracentesis, open lung biopsy, subTAH, BSO, (Depo-Provera)	Catamenial hemothorax, pelvic endometriosis, severe
Rosenberg, 1981 [36]	37	Hemoptysis	Symptoms concurrent with menses	Unknown	Bronchoscopy, (danazol)	Catamenial hemoptysis, pelvic endometriosis
Wilhelm, 1977 [37]	32	Right shoulder pain, substernal chest pain, dyspnea, bilateral pneumothorax	Symptoms concurrent with menses, severe dysmenorrhea	Unknown	Thoracentesis right exploratory thoractomy, abrasive pleurodesis (Ovral, Depo-Provera)	Catamenial hemoptysis, pleural endometriosis
Grandberg, 1977 [38]	35	Chest pain	Symptoms concurrent with menses	Previous cesarean, resection of ovarian cyst, left ovariectomy	Aspiration biopsy of the right lung, diagnostic pneumothorax, thoracoscopy (mestranol-noretisteron)	Pulmonary endometriosis, pelvic endometriosis

Endometriosis of the appendix is somewhat less common than that of the large bowel and rectum but shares an equal incidence with endometriosis of the small bowel. Of the same 35 cases of intestinal endometriosis (Table III), 6 involved the appendix and, of this number, 50% included intussusception of the appendix. All of these women required appendectomy and/or hemicolectomy. Endometriosis of the small bowel and omentum were so infrequent that diagnosis and treatment would be dependent upon the location and the extent of the disease. Although hormonal therapy is usually ineffective, a recent report suggests omental endometriosis may respond to suppressive therapy with medroxyprogesterone [24]. Surgical excision should be reserved for failed responses to suppressive therapy.

Urinary Tract Endometriosis

Urinary tract endometriosis may be divided into involvement of the bladder wall, ureter, and kidneys. Whereas Williams and Pratt [25] found small or large bowel involvement in 33% of a group of women with pelvic endometriosis, they only found urinary involvement in 16% of the same group. In the majority of these women, urinary tract endometriosis consisted of implants on the peritoneal surface of the bladder. Only 1.5% exhibited ureteral involvement. The bladder lesions may be of superficial involvement or may penetrate more deeply into the muscular layer. The superficial bladder endometriosis is best explained by implantation after retrograde menstruation similar to that involving the uterus, tubes, ovaries, and overlying pelvic peritoneum. Endometriosis extending into the muscular coat would likely occur as a result of direct infiltration.

Ureteral endometriosis may develop through direct involvement from endometriosis occurring within the muscle wall or by indirect involvement of adjacent organs, particularly the uterosacral ligament and/or ovary. Ureteral involvement commonly leads to obstruction resulting in pain, dysuria, hematuria, hydronephrosis, or pyelonephritis. It is common for the symptoms of pain, dysuria, and hematuria to occur in a cyclic fashion relating to menstrual periods. Involvement of the kidneys with endometriosis is extremely rare but should be included in a differential diagnosis of patients presenting with cyclic lumbar pain and hematuria (Table IV).

Our treatment of ureteral and bladder endometriosis depends on the extent and location of disease, age of the patient, and degree of symptoms. Conservative therapy with hormonal suppression has been successful. However, in most cases of ureter obstruction, surgical therapy is indicated and would include a total abdominal hysterectomy and bilateral salpingo-oophorectomy when fertility is no longer desired. Correction of obstruction may be accomplished by ureteral diversion, reimplantation, or reanastomosis. Bladder lesions are managed by hormonal suppression or local excision and/or fulguration. In some women, mucosal involvement will require segmental resection of a portion of the bladder wall.

Endometriosis in Other Sites

Aside from extra pelvic endometriosis involving the intestinal tract, the urinary tract, and the lung, endometriosis has been reported as occurring in virtually every portion of the body. Recent literature had indicated involvement in the vagina, Bartholin's and Skein's glands, urethra, episiotomy site, vulva, abdominal incisions, umbilicus, pancreas, nerves, and extremities (Table IV). Of these locations, endometriosis of the umbilicus seems to be the most common and presents with pain and a palpable mass in the umbilical area. Of interest have been two recent cases of endometriosis of the pancreas, which presented in one case with left flank pain and a palpable mass and in the other case with epigastric pain and right upper quadrant fullness [26,27]. Both were treated surgically with a distal pancreatectomy and splenectomy

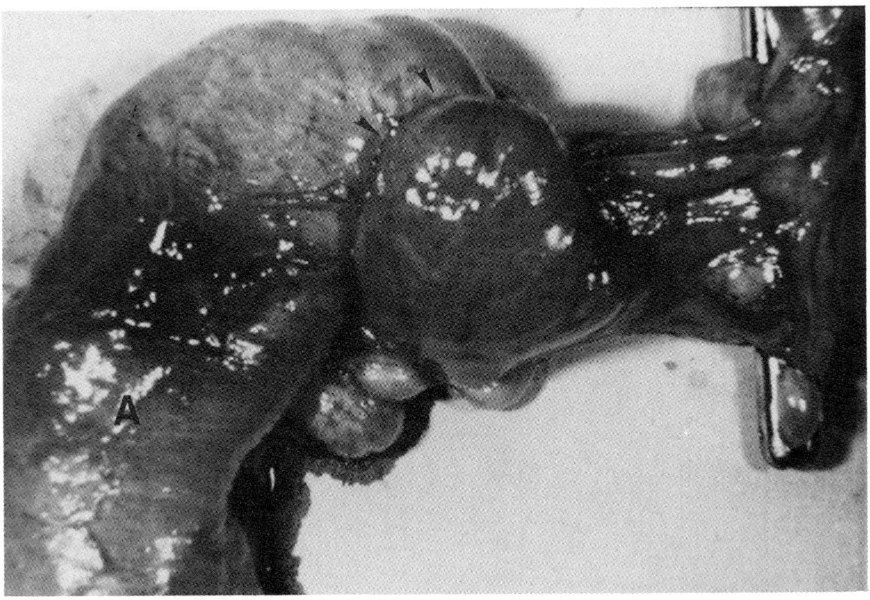

Fig. 3. Endometriosis of the sigmoid colon demonstrating subserosal implants (**A**) and partial obstruction requiring resection.

TABLE III. Clinical Data - Intestinal/Omental Endometriosis

Author	Age	Bowel symptoms	Gynecologic symptoms	Previous OB/GYN surgery	Operative procedure	Diagnosis
Thiel, 1986 [39]	41	Abdominal and back pain, vomiting	Asymptomatic pelvic	None	Drainage of right ovarian cyst, partial right hemi-colectomy	Endometriosis of the appendix and cecum
Narayn-singh, 1985 [24]	24	Abdominal distension and discomfort	Dysmenorrhea	None	Paracentesis, biopsy of omentum (Depo-Provera)	Omental endometriosis with ascites
Mann, 1984 [40]	41	None	Abnormal uterine bleeding, dysmenorrhea, and dyspareunia	Tubal ligation and D&Cs	Abdominal hysterectomy, and left salpingo-oophorectomy and appendectomy	Leiomyomas endometrial cyst of left ovary, appendix with intus-susception and endometriosis
	58	Ascites	Pelvic mass	TAH and bilateral salpingo-oophorectomy, omentectomy	Resection and appendectomy	Recurrent endometri-od carcinoma and appendix with intussusception and endometriosis
Floberg, 1984 [41]	34	Pain in right lower quadrant	Pregnancy, postpartum	None	Resection of left ovarian abscess and segment of sigmoid	Colon endometriosis and perforation
Caccese, 1984 [42]	37	Recurrent rectal bleeding	None	None	Flexible sigmoidoscopy	Endometriosis of the colon
Langsam, 1984 [43]	32	Low abdominal pain with nausea and vomiting	Symptoms worse at menses	None	Colotomy with appendectomy, excision of left ovarian endometrioma	Pelvic endometriosis appendix with endo-metriosis and intus-susception
Hardy, 1983 [44]	40	Midabdominal pain, dis-tension, vomiting and diarrhea	None	None	Resection of terminal ileum and cecum	Endometriosis of the terminal ileum

Forsgren, 1983 [22]	43	Obstruction and diarrhea	None	Unknown	Anterior resection of the colon	Endometriosis of the colon and rectum
	40	Obstruction and pain	None	Unknown	Colpotomy and laparotomy	Endometriosis of the colon and rectum
	51	Obstruction	None	Unknown	Laparotomy and dissection of sigmoid obstruction	Endometriosis of the colon and rectum
	45	Obstruction, pain, diarrhea	None	Unknown	Anterior resection	Endometriosis of the colon and rectum
	40	Obstruction, rectal bleeding	Symptoms worse at menses	Unknown	Laparoscopy	Endometriosis of the colon and rectum
	40	Obstruction and pain	Symptoms worse at menses	Unknown	Laparotomy and dissection of rectal obstruction	Endometriosis of the colon and rectum
Teunen, 1982 [13]	47	Diarrhea and constipation	None	Unknown	Oophorectomy	Endometriosis of the anterior rectal wall
	29	None	Infertility	Unknown	Resection of endometriosis	Endometriosis of the rectosigmoidal area
	47	(Increased urinary frequency)	None	Unknown	Resection of endometriosis	Endometriosis of the rectosigmoidal area
	60	Right lower quadrant pain	None	Unknown	None	Endometriosis of the rectosigmoidal area
	33	None	Dysmenorrhea and menometrorrhagia	Unknown	None (progestagens)	Endometriosis of the sigmoid colon
	47	Constipation	Dysmenorrhea	Unknown	None	Endometriosis of the sigmoid colon
	38	None	Dysmenorrhea and menometrorrhagia	Unknown	Resection of endometriosis	Endometriosis of the sigmoid colon
	48	Constipation, right lower quadrant pain (renal insufficiency)	Menometrorrhagia	Unknown	Presacral neurectomy (progestagens, urine deviation)	Endometriosis of the sigmoid colon
	37	Left lower quadrant pain, diarrhea, constipation, hematochezia	Secondary infertility	Unknown	Resection of endometriosis (danazol and progestagens)	Endometriosis of the sigmoid colon

(continued)

TABLE III. Clinical Data - Intestinal/Omental Endometriosis (continued)

Author	Age	Bowel symptoms	Gynecologic symptoms	Previous OB/GYN surgery	Operative procedure	Diagnosis
	40	Left lower quadrant pain, diarrhea, constipation, hematochezia	None	Unknown	Resection of endometriosis (progestagens)	Endometriosis of the sigmoid colon
	41	Constipation, hematochezia	None	Unknown	(progestagens)	Endometriosis of the sigmoid colon
	41	Constipation, diarrhea	Dysmenorrhea	Unknown	(progestagens)	Endometriosis of the sigmoid colon
	38	Left lower quadrant pain, hematochezia	Infertility, dysmenorrhea	Unknown	Resection of endometriosis	Endometriosis of the sigmoid colon
	33	None	Infertility	Unknown	Appendectomy	Endometriosis of the appendix and ileum
	28	None	Dysmenorrhea, infertility	Unknown	Ileocecal resection	Endometriosis of the ileocecal area, appendix, and ascending colon
	39	Diarrhea, hematochezia	Infertility	Unknown	Resection of endometriosis (progestagens)	Endometriosis of the ileum
	33	None	Infertility	Unknown	Resection of endometriosis (progestagens)	Endometriosis of the ileum
	45	Right lower quadrant pain, cyclic small bowel obstruction	None	Unknown	Ileocecal resection	Endometriosis of the ileocecal angle
Farinon, 1980 [45]	42	None	Multiple uterine fibroids	Unknown	Hysterectomy and left salpingo-oophorectomy	Endometriosis of the rectum
	41	None	Uterine fibroma	Unknown	Hysterectomy and left salpingo-oophorectomy (progestagens)	Endometriosis of the rectosigmoid colon
	36	Pelvic pain	None	Unknown	Myomectomy, left oophorectomy (progestagens)	Endometriosis of the left ovary and the sigmoid colon (fibroma of the uterus)

plus, in one case, a radical left nephrectomy. Our treatment of endometriosis of other sites is dependent totally upon the location and the extent of lesion, but most commonly involves excision of the ectopic endometrium, with or without hormonal suppression.

COMMENT

Endometriosis can occur in almost every organ of the body. This diagnosis should always be considered when symptoms of pain and/or a palpable mass or lesion occurs in a cyclic sequence with menses. Even though extra pelvic or nongynecologic endometriosis is statistically an uncommon lesion, its frequency has been reported in increasing numbers and, as a result, in the practice of gynecology its importance has increased. Of the nongynecologic sites in which endometriosis has been reported, the intestinal tract, specifically the large bowel and rectum, have been most common. Additionally, endometriosis of the lung, with involvement of the pleura as well as the parenchyma, has been recorded and represents the second most common site outside of the pelvic organs. Involvement of the urinary tract does occur with sufficient frequency but probably is the result of extension of endometriosis of the pelvic organs. Endometriosis has additionally been found in the thumb, the knee, the sciatic nerve, the thigh, the umbilicus, the vulva, the vagina, the cervix, and in incisional scars of the abdomen and the perineum. Diagnosis and treatment of intestinal tract endometriosis depends on the location, the extent of disease, and symptoms resulting from the involvement as well as the desire for continued fertility. Surgery has been reported as the most successful therapy. However, treatment with hormones such as danazol or medroxyprogesterone has been successful in cases of less severe involvement and in those patients in whom significant obstruction has not occurred.

Pulmonary endometriosis has generally presented with either hemothorax, pneumothorax, or hemoptysis occurring at the time of menses or, in a small number of cases, with pulmonary lesions or nodules. Over 90% of all cases occurred in the right chest. In cases of catamenial hemothorax and pneumothorax, occurrence with pelvic endometriosis was common, whereas with catamential hemoptysis such a relationship does not exist. Successful therapy of pulmonary endometriosis more commonly occurred with surgical intervention including thorocotomy, pleurodesis, excision of endometriotic nodules, and implants and closure of diaphragmatic defects. Recent literature, as well as personal experience, supports the benefits of suppressive therapy with danazol or medroxyprogesterone, although medical literature during the last 6 years continues to support surgery as the most beneficial form of therapy in women who wish to conserve ovarian function.

TABLE IV. Clinical Data - Urinary Tract Endometriosis

Author	Age	Urinary tract symptoms	Gynecologic symptoms	Previous OB/GYN surgery	Operative procedure	Diagnosis
Porena, 1985 [46]	54	Microhematuria, left flank pain	None	None	Nephroureterectomy, excision of lymph node	Endometriosis of the ureter
Plous, 1985 [47]	74	Dysuria, frequency, hematuria	None	None	Ureteral resection and implantation	Endometriosis of the ureter
Matsuura, 1985 [48]	21	Increasing body weight	Dysmenorrhea	None	Left salpingo-oophorectomy, biopsy of pelvic and abdominal endometriosis (danazol)	Endometriosis of the pelvis and ureter
Vermesh, 1985 [49]	39	Intermittent hematuria, dysuria, frequency, urgency	None	Vaginal hysterectomy	Excision of endometriosis	Endometriosis of the bladder wall
Gantt, 1980 [50]	26	Low abdominal pain	Symptoms worse with menses	None	Laparotomy with resection of ovarian endometriomas (Depo-Provera)	Pelvic endometriosis with endometriosis of the ureter
Moore, 1979 [51]	43	Backache	Dysmenorrhea	None	TAH, BSO, resection of the distal third of the left ureter, left ureteroneocystotomy	Pelvic endometriosis with endometriosis of the left ureter
	30	None	Pelvic mass	None	TAH, BSO, left ureteral lysis	Pelvic endometriosis

32	Premenstrual dysuria	Dysmenorrhea	None	TAH, BSO, bilateral ureteral lysis	Pelvic endometriosis with endometriosis of both ureters
25	Flank pain, hematuria	Dysmenorrhea	None	TAH, BSO, and right ureteroneocystotomy	Pelvic endometriosis with endometriosis of the right ureter
33	Left hydro-nephrosis	Dyspareunia, pelvic mass	None	Resection of left kidney and ureter, resection of pelvic endometriosis	Pelvic endometriosis with endometriosis of left pelvic wall involving left ureter
26	Dysuria with menses	Dysmenorrhea with lower left quadrant pain	None	Open resection of the bladder, segmental resection of colon, right ureteral lysis	Pelvic endometriosis with endometriosis of bladder wall, omentum
44	None	Right lower quadrant pain	Right salpingo-oophorectomy, total abdominal hysterectomy, left salpingo-oophorectomy	Proximal right ureter ostomy, ureteral lysis, resection of bladder wall endometriosis	Pelvic endometriosis with endometriosis of bladder and right ureter
21	Impaired drainage of right ureter	Dysmenorrhea	None	Right ureterolysis, resection of endometrioma of uterosacral ligament	Pelvic endometriosis with endometriosis of right uterosacral ligament

TABLE V. Clinical Data – Endometriosis of Other Sites

Author	Age	Presenting symptoms	Gynecologic symptoms	Previous OB/GYN surgery	Operative procedure	Diagnosis
Goswami, 1985 [27]	40	Left flank pain, palpable 'renal' mass	None	None	Radical left nephrectomy, distal pancreatectomy splenectomy	Pancreatic endometriosis
Marchevsky, 1984 [26]	36	Epigastric pain, right lower quadrant fullness, left lower quadrant tenderness	None	None	Laparotomy with distal pancreatectomy and splenectomy	Pancreatic endometriosis
Gupta, 1985 [5]	42	Pain and bleeding from left thumb	Symptoms only during menses	None	Wide excision of lesion	Endometriosis of the tip of the thumb
Patel, 1982 [52]	32	Painful swelling of the knee	None	Laparoscopic tubal sterilization	(Danazol) following biopsy	Endometriosis of the knee
Gitelis, 1985 [31]	31	Painful soft tissue mass	Symptoms increased with menses	None	Excision of mass from right thigh	Endometriosis of the thigh

Pellegrini, 1981 [53]	36	Intermittent pain in right groin, tenderness in the external inguinal	Tender mass overlying pubic tubercle	None	Excision of mass	Endometrioma of the pubis
	30	Intermittent pain in right groin and hip	Symptoms worse just before menses	None	Excision of mass	Endometrioma
Hibbard, 1984 [8]	40	Right footdrop, right hip pain	Pelvic endometriosis	Total abdominal hysterectomy, right salpingo-oophorectomy	Exploration of the right sciatic nerve, biopsy and lysis of adhesions, LSO, (Provera)	Endometriosis of the sciatic nerve
Brzezinski, 1983 [54]	41	Right inguinal mass with pain	Symptoms worse during menses	None	Excision of mass in right indirect hernia sac	Endometriosis of connective tissue in a hernia sac
Michowitz, 1983 [14]	43	Periumbilical pain with mass	None	None	Excision of umbilical mass	Endometriosis of the umbilicus
Blumenthal 1981 [55]	46	Lump in the umbilicus with pain	Symptoms worse during menses	None	Excision of umbilical mass	Endometriosis of the umbilicus

Urinary endometriosis, though less common, is of special significance because of ureteral obstruction. In such cases, surgical intervention, including ureteral reimplantation or anastomosis is indicated. Endometriosis of other extra pelvic sites has been recorded, though infrequently, in virtually every area of the body. As these women are frequently symptomatic at the time of menses, the physician should include endometriosis as a possible etiologic factor in differential diagnosis of symptoms or lesions that follow a cyclic pattern related to the menses. Therapy of distant site disease would depend on the extent of the disease, but should include local excision and/or hormonal suppression. Occasionally, castration is indicated in such patients and then only when fertility is no longer desired.

REFERENCES

1. Saleh N, Daw E: Endometriosis in non-gynecological sites. Practitioner 224:1189, 1980.
2. Lane RE: Endometriosis of the vermiform appendix. J Obstet Gynecol 79:372, 1960.
3. Goodman JD, Macchia RJ, Macasaet MA, Schneider M: Endometriosis of the urinary bladder. Am J Radiol 135:625, 1980.
4. Williams JF, Richardson AC: Endometriosis of cervix uteri. Obstet Gynecol 6:309, 1955.
5. Gupta SD: Endometriosis in the thumb. J Indian M A 83:122, 1985.
6. Novak ER, Jones GS, Jones HW: Endometriosis. In Novak ER, Jones GS, Jones HW Jr, (eds): "Novak's Textbook of Gynecology," 8th ed. Baltimore: Williams & Wilkins, pp 474–494, 1970.
7. Strasser EJ, Davis EM: Extraperitoneal inguinal endometriosis. Am Surg 43:421, 1977.
8. Hibbard J, Schreiber JR: Footdrop due to sciatic nerve endometriosis. Am J Obstet Gynecol 149:800, 1984.
9. Foster DC, Stern JL, Buscema J, Rock JA, Woodruff JD: Pleural and parenchymal pulmonary endometriosis. Obstet Gynecol 58:552, 1981.
10. Hawthorne HR, Kimbrough RA, David HC: Concomitant endometriosis and carcinoma of the rectosigmoid. Am J Obstet Gynecol 62:681, 1951.
11. Javert CT: Spread of benign and malignant endometrium in the lymphatic system. Am J Obstet Gynecol 64:780, 1952.
12. Meyers WC, Kelvin FM, Jones RS: Diagnosis and surgical treatment of colonic endometriosis. Arch Surg 114:169, 1979.
13. Teunen A, Ooms ECM, Tytgat GNJ: Endometriosis of the samll and large bowel. Neth J Med 25:142, 1982.
14. Michowitz M, Baratz M, Stavorovsky M: Endometriosis of the umbilicus. Dermatologica 167:326, 1983.
15. Duson CK, Zelenik JS: Vulvar endometriosis. Obstet Gynecol 3:76, 1954.
16. Barbieri R, Kistner RW: Endometriosis. In Kistner RW, (ed): "Gynecology: Principles and Practice," 4th ed. Chicago: Year Book Medical Publishers, pp 393–414, 1986.
17. Meigs JV: The medical treatment of endometriosis and The significance of endometriosis. Surg Gynecol Obstet 89:317, 1949.
18. Williams TJ: Endometriosis. In Mattingly RF, Thompson JD (eds): "TeLinde's Operative Gynecology," 6th ed. Philadelphia: J.B. Lippincott, pp 257–286, 1985.

19. Yates-Bell AL, Molland EA, Pryor JP: Endometriosis of the ureter. Br J Urol 44:58, 1972.
20. Ball TL, Platt MA: Urologic complications of endometriosis. Am J Obstet Gynecol 84:1516, 1962.
21. Karpel P, Appel D, Merav A: Pulmonary endometriosis. Lung 163:151, 1985.
22. Forsgren H, Lindhagen J, Melander S, Wagermark J: Colorectal endometriosis. Acta Chir Scand 149:431, 1983.
23. Macafee CH, Greer HL: Intestinal endometriosis. A report of 29 cases and a survey of the literature. J Obstet gynecol Br Emp 67:538, 1960.
24. Naraynsingh V, Raju GC, Ratan P, Wong J: Massive ascites due to omental endometriosis. Postgrad Med J 61:539, 1985.
25. Williams TJ, Pratt JH: Endometriosis in 1,000 consecutive celiotomies: incidence and management. Am J Obstet Gynecol 129:245, 1977.
26. Marchevsky AM, Zimmerman MJ, Aufses AH, Weiss H: Endometrial cyst of the pancreas. Gastroenterology 86:1589, 1984.
27. Goswami AK, Sharma SK, Tandon SP, et al.: Pancreatic endometriosis presenting as a hypovascular renal mass. J Urol 135:112, 1986.
28. Ranney B: Endometriosis: pathogenesis, symptoms and findings. Clin Obstet Gynecol 23:865, 1980.
29. Meyers WC, Kelvin FM, Jones RS: Diagnosis and surgical treatment of colonic endometriosis. Arch Surg 114:169, 1979.
30. Meigs JV: Endometriosis: its significance. Ann Surg 114:866, 1941.
31. Gitelis S, Petasnick JP, Turner DA, Ghiselli RW, Miller AW: Endometriosis stimulating a soft tissue tumor of the thigh: CT and MR evaluation. J Comput Assist Tomogr 9:573, 1985.
32. Scott RB, TeLinde RW: External endometriosis: the scourge of the private patient. Ann Surg 131:697, 1950.
33. Suginami H, Hamada K, Yano K: A case of endometriosis of the lung treated with danazol. Obstet Gynecol 66:68S(supplement), 1985.
34. Wilkins SB, Bell-Thompson J, Tyras DH: Hemothorax associated with endometriosis. J Thorac Cardiovasc Surg 89:636, 1985.
35. Hibbard LT, Schumann WR, Goldstein GE: Thoracic endometriosis: a review and report of two cases. Am J Obstet Gynecol 140:227, 1981.
36. Rosenberg SM, Riddick DH: Successful treatment of catamenial hemoptysis with danazol. Obstet Gynecol 57:130, 1981.
37. Wilhelm JL, Scommegna A: Catamenial pneumothorax. Obstet Gynecol 50:227, 1977.
38. Grandberg I, Willems JS: Endometriosis of lung and pleura diagnosed by aspiration biopsy. Acta Cytol 21:295, 1977.
39. Thiel CW: Endometriosis of the cecum associated with appendicitis. Minnesota Med 69:20, 1986.
40. Mann WJ, Fromowitz F, Sayshek T, Madariaga JR, Chalas E: Endometriosis associated with appendiceal intussusception. J Reprod Med 29:625, 1984.
41. Floberg J, Backdahl M, Silfersward C, Thomassen PA: Postpartum perforation of the colon due to endometriosis. Acta Obstet Gynecol Scand 63:183, 1984.
42. Caccese WJ, McKinley MJ, Bronzo RL, Bronson R: Endoscopic confirmation of colonic endometriosis. Gastrointest Endosc 30:191, 1984.
43. Langsam LB, Raj PK, Galang CF: Intussusception of the appendix. Dis Colon Rectum 27:387, 1984.

44. Hardy RF, Kaude JV: Invasive endometriosis of the terminal ileum: a cause of small bowel obstruction of obscure origin. South Med J 76:253, 1983.
45. Farinon AM, Vadora E: Endometriosis of the colon and rectum: an indication for preoperative colonoscopy. Endoscopy 12:136, 1980.
46. Porena M, Vespasiani G, Virgili G, Mearini E, Micali F: Ureteral endometriosis: an endoscopic diagnosis. Urology 26:566, 1985.
47. Plous RH, Sunshine R, Goldman H, Schwartz IS: Ureteral endometriosis in post-menopausal women. Urology 26:408, 1985.
48. Matsuura K, Kawasaki N, Oka M, Maeyama H, Maeyama M: Treatment with danazol of ureteral obstruction caused by endometriosis. Acta Obstet Gynecol Scand 64:339, 1985.
49. Vermesh M, Zbella EA, Menchaca A, Confino E, Lipshitz S: Vesical endometriosis following bladder injury. Am J Obstet Gynecol 153:894, 1985.
50. Gantt PA, Hunt JB, McDonough PG: Progestin reversal of ureteral endometriosis. Obstet Gynecol 57:665, 1981.
51. Moore JG, Hibbard LT, Growdon WA, Schifrin BS: Urinary tract endometriosis: enigmas in diagnosis and management. Am J Obstet Gynecol 134:162, 1979.
52. Patel VC, Samuels H, Abeles E, Hirjibehedin PF: Endometriosis at the knee. Clin Ortho 171:140, 1982.
53. Pellegrini VD, Pasternak HS, Maculay WP: Endometrioma of the pubis: a differential in the diagnosis of hip pain. J Bone Joint Surg 63A:1333, 1981.
54. Brzezinski A, Durst AL: Endometriosis presenting as an inguinal hernia. Am J Obstet Gynecol 146:982, 1983.
55. Blumenthal NJ: Umbilical endometriosis. S Afr Med J 59:198, 1981.

Endometriosis, pages 207–223

Chapter 12
Experimental Endometriosis

Michael W. Vernon, Ph.D., and Gary D. Hodgen, Ph.D.

Kentucky Center for Reproductive Medicine, Department of Obstetrics and Gynecology, University of Kentucky Medical Center, Lexington, Kentucky 40536 (M.W.V.) and Eastern Virginia Medical School, Jones Institute for Reproductive Medicine, Department of Obstetrics and Gynecology, Norfolk, Virginia 23507

INTRODUCTION

The presence of endometrial tissue outside of the lumen of the uterus was first reported almost 300 years ago by Saviard, in 1696 [1]. Since the turn of the century it has been known that these ectopic loci of endometrial tissue were responsible for dysmenorrhea, dyspareunia, pain on defecation [2,3], and more recently for infertility [4]. Even though endometriosis has been well described and its symptomology known for over 50 years, our current appreciation of the pathophysiological mechanisms of this disease is still unclear. The principal reasons for this lack of information are 1) most patients who present with endometriosis have had the disease for an extended period of time, and 2) endometriosis occurs naturally in only humans and nonhuman primates [5]. The first factor makes it difficult to initiate any clinical experiments that would definitively determine the etiology or progression of the disease, and owing to the ethical considerations of the second factor, properly controlled or invasive experiments cannot be performed. Because of these factors, there has been an obvious need for the development of techniques for the induction of endometriosis in research animals. Surgical induction of the disease in animals would allow for the construction of controlled experiments on the etiology, development, and endocrine interrelationships of endometriosis.

If the symptoms of endometriosis are a result of the ectopic nature of the endometriotic implant, then the surgical attachment of endometrium to the viscera of research animals could serve as a model for endometriosis. The ability of epithelial tissue, and in particular endometrial tissue, to proliferate after autotransplantation to various ectopic locations is not a new observation. In 1903, Stilling found that pieces of uterine and vaginal tissue collected from immature rabbits would continue to grow when transplanted to the spleen of the same animal [6]. These implants grew into large cystic formations that were filled with a clear or mottled secretion. In 1905, Nichols published an extensive study on the etiology of cancer in which he reported the transplantation of portions of various organs, including the uterus, to numerous locations within the bodies of rabbits and guinea-pigs. The subcutaneous transplantation of strips of uterine tissue to the abdomen grew into "cystic-like tumors" that were lined with endometrial epithelium [7].

With the suggestion by Sampson in the 1920's that endometriosis was due to reverse regurgitation of menstrual components into the peritoneal cavity [8,9], Jacobson attempted the first surgical procedures for the purpose of developing an animal model for endometriosis [10,11]. In support of Sampson's theory, all endometrial tissue that he autotransplanted to the peritoneal cavity of the rabbit [10] and monkey [11] were found to grow in a fashion similar to the human disease.

The ease with which ectopic endometrial tissue proliferates within the peritoneal cavity of research animals is not, in itself, sufficient evidence for the use of animals as research models for endometriosis. In order for induced endometriosis to function as a model of the disease, the model must evoke the symptoms of endometriosis. The two prominent symptoms of endometriosis are pain (e.g., dysmenorrhea and dyspareunia) and infertility.The measurement of pain in animals is difficult to assess and at best can only be qualitatively measured. However, the influence of endometriosis upon fertility can be easily quantified and has recently been studied in the monkey [12], rat [13], and rabbit [14]. In all three species a reduction in the fecundity of the animal was observed as a consequence of surgical induction of endometriosis. Thus research animals with surgically induced endometriosis appear to have some of the symptoms of human endometriosis and, subsequently, have the potential of serving as models for studying those aspects of the disease that cannot be adequately investigated in the human. The intent of the remainder of this chapter is, therefore, to delineate the surgical procedures required to induce endometriosis in the monkey, rat, and rabbit and to present the current status of endometriosis research in these species.

SURGICAL INDUCTION OF ENDOMETRIOSIS IN THE MONKEY

Reproductive Endocrinology

The two most commonly used old world monkeys that have been utilized for laboratory work and for the surgical induction of endometriosis are the rhesus (*Macaca mulatta*) and the cynomolgus or crab-eating monkey (*Ma-*

caca fascicularis). These monkeys have a 28-day menstrual cycle that is endocrinologically similar to the human, with ovulation occurring between days 12 to 15 after the onset of menstruation [15]. The majority of monkeys housed in a vivarium will have menstrual cycles throughout the year; however, the monkey is considered a seasonal breeder with its time of high fecundity occurring during fall and early winter [16]. The reproductive cycle of the monkey can be easily documented with daily monitoring for menstrual flow and changes in the color intensity (red) and turgescence of the perineal skin [17]. A more exact method of assessing cyclicity can also be obtained by monitoring the cytology of vaginal lavages [18] or by measuring plasma estrogen and progesterone and urinary LH concentrations.

Methodology

Endometriosis occurs spontaneously in the nonhuman primate [19,20] and as such has been suggested and used as a model for the human disease by MacKenzie [20]. While less than 1% of rhesus breeders have been reported to be afflicted with spontaneous disease [20], underreporting and lack of clinical follow-up for infertility makes us highly skeptical that the real occurrence rate is appreciated. Nevertheless, this low rate of availability of monkeys with spontaneous endometriosis curtails their experimental use. The method of choice for using the monkey as a model for endometriosis has been through the surgical introduction of the disease.

Experimental endometriosis has been readily introduced into monkeys by implantation of autologous endometrial tissue to the abdominal cavity (Fig. 1). Three methods of surgically inducing the disease have been successfully employed: 1) diverting the cervix from the vagina to the peritoneal cavity [21], 2) suturing segments of endometrial tissue to the peritoneal cavity [11,22], and 3) seeding the peritoneal cavity with minced fragments of endometrium [23].

Experimental Observations

Jacobson [11] was the first to use the monkey model, in 1926, three years after he introduced the concept of utilizing an animal model by inducing endometriosis in the rabbit [10]. Although Jacobson indicated a high success rate for inducing the disease in the monkey, very few experiments were performed with this model until TeLinde and Scott rekindled an interest in the model in the 1950's [21].

To assess the viability of menstrual fragments and to validate the retrograde theory of Sampson [8,9], TeLinde and Scott [21] developed a procedure that was designed to permit intraabdominal menstruation. The cervix of 10 mon-

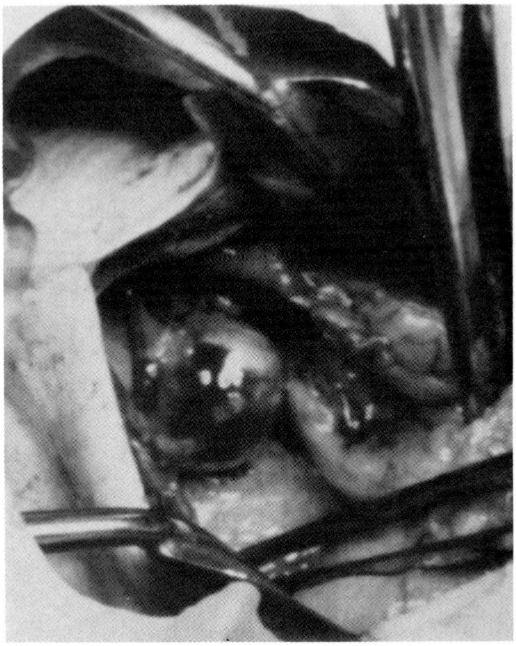

Fig. 1. Surgically exposed abdominal viscera of the monkey showing the appearance of endometriotic implants after surgical autotransplantation of endometrial tissue (photo courtesy of Dr. Robert S. Schenken).

keys were surgically diverted to the abdominal cavity. Five of these animals developed severe adhesions that were histologically confirmed to contain endometrial tissue. Most of the disease was confined to the area of the os cervix; however, one monkey developed gross and microscopic endometriosis on the bowel wall and the pelvic peritoneum. These data confirmed the ability of "cast-off" menstrual components to be viable and capable of implantation. They were also interpreted as offering additional support for the retrograde theory of Sampson [9]. Several individuals during this time period were skeptical of TeLinde and Scott's interpretations, because it was felt that endometrial cells may have been liberated during the surgical procedure and that monkey experiments could not be extrapolated to human pathology. To answer this question Ridley and Edwards injected human menstrual components into the peritoneum of eight women [24]. Menstrual fluid was collected in a sterile fashion as it flowed from the cervix, and the menstrual detritus was separated from the blood and injected through an 18-gauge needle onto the abdominal fascia. Two of the patients developed scar tissue, and one of these patients contained endometriosis, which was confirmed by histological analysis [24]. Although studies of this nature cannot be performed by today's code of ethics, these studies present parallels between the monkey model and human endometriosis that support the use of research animals as models for controlled experiments that cannot be ethically conducted with humans.

The major emphasis of current experiments with the monkey model has been directed at the role of steroids in controlling the growth and development of endometriotic implants. The obligatory role of steroid stimulation on implant proliferation in the human can be inferred by the remission of symptoms and regression of implant after ovariectomy or menopause. Scott and Wharton attempted to identify the role of steroid modulation of implant growth in 13 ovariectomized monkeys by administering either no hormone, constant estrone or progesterone, or constant estrone with intermittent progesterone to mimic the cycle [22]. This experimental paradigm was proposed in an attempt not only to assess steroid requirements but also to confirm whether progesterone withdrawal from estrogen stimulation would result in "menstruation" from endometriotic implants. After as much as 37 months of this exogenous hormone treatment, viable implants were noted in at least one animal from each group. However, the implants from the intermittent progesterone treatment were two to three times larger than those found in animals subjected to constant steroid. Old or recent hemorrhage areas were evident in implants from all treatment groups but not in the steroid-deficient animals, leading the authors to suggest that implants may function as "miniature uteri." Although the implants may have shed endometrial components, no implant dissemination to areas other than the original surgical sites were observed. The steroid-dependent nature of endometriotic implants has also been recently examined by Dizerega and coworkers [23]. Castrated monkeys received subcutaneous capsules containing no hormone, estradiol, progesterone, or estradiol plus progesterone for 4, 12, or 16 weeks. Endometriotic implants were found in all groups at 4 weeks, but after that period implants in the control animals underwent regression and were found only to contain "burnt-out" plaques. The authors concluded that autotransplanted endometrial tissue required no steroid supplementation for initiation of implantation but that subsequent growth was steroid dependent [23].

Because pregnancy was shown to have beneficial effects upon endometriosis, several therapies using progestins and diethystilbestrol (DES) were devised from 1950 to 1960. These drugs were shown, at that time, to be effective in relieving the symptoms of endometriosis and enhancing the patient's fertility rate [25,26]. The efficacy of treating endometriosis with synthetic progestins [27] and DES [28] was examined in the monkey model by Scott and Wharton. These drugs were found to maintain implant size in a fashion similar to that observed previously with progesterone and estrogen treatments. However, the progestin, norethindrone, did evoke moderate necrosis of the stromal cells of implants and uteri [27] and DES induced uterine and implant epithelial hyperplasia [28]. As a secondary observation, Scott and Wharton histologically examined the pelvic lymph nodes of four animals receiving DES and noted the presence of endometrial glands in all four animals [28].

As noted by Dizerega and coworkers [23], these data present a paradoxical observation. Endometriotic implants appear to thrive under steroid exposure, yet symptomatology is arrested in humans, receiving estrogen/progestin therapies. However, the beneficial effect of the contraceptive pill may be due to the cessation of menstrual cycles, which would prevent retrograde menstruation and progression of the disease. Alternately, as suggested by Scott and Wharton [22], cyclicity of hormones may predispose the implant to grow while the absence of hormone cycles leads to implant maintenance without growth.

To assess the endocrine mechanisms whereby endometriosis reduces fertility, Schenken and coworkers [12] characterized the hormonal cycles and fecundity of 21 monkeys with and without surgically induced endometriosis. The extent of the disease within these animals was classified according to the guidelines of the American Fertility Society [29], and the status of the ovulatory phase ovary and peritoneal cavity was assessed by laparoscopy. Monkeys with moderate and severe endometriosis had lower chemical and term pregnancy rates than control animals. Luteinized unruptured follicles (LUFS) were observed in five of ten cycles in monkeys with moderate endometriosis and three of six with severe disease, whereas LUFS were absent in control animals. Furthermore, the presence of adhesions ipsolateral to the side of the ovulating ovary completely prevented conception. The authors concluded that the impaired fertility of monkeys with induced endometriosis appeared to be mediated primarily by failure of follicular rupture and/or pelvic adhesions [12].

Summary

The monkey represents a suitable animal for the study of endometriosis, because it has a menstrual cycle similar to the human and is known to be afflicted with spontaneous endometriosis. Furthermore, the high success rate of surgically inducing the disease and the marked similarity between the gross and histological appearance of the monkey model to the human disease also adds to the appeal of the monkey model. However, the high cost and the intense maintenance problems associated with the monkey limit the use of these species for many laboratories.

SURGICAL INDUCTION OF ENDOMETRIOSIS IN THE RAT

Reproductive Endocrinology

The laboratory rat (*Rattus norvegicus*) is a polytoccus mammal that exhibits a 4- to 5-day estrous cycle. Puberty occurs within 2 months of birth, and the reproductive life of the rat lasts for approximately 1.5 to 2 years. The highly predictable reproductive cycle of the rat has been exhaustively studied and can be reliably monitored with daily vaginal lavages. The reproductive endocrine pattern of the rat follows the same temporal sequence as the human. The major deviation between the rat and human is the duration of the luteral phase of the cycle, which is shorter in the rat. The reproductive cycle of the rat is extremely sensitive to photoperiod, and animals must be housed in a 14:10 hr or 12:12 hr (light:dark) lighting regime in order to maintain their estrous cycles. Constant light or a short burst of light during the dark period will induce a period of constant estrus that may last for several weeks.

Methodology

The method of choice for the surgical induction of endometriosis in the rat has been through the autotransplantation of uterine squares to the peritoneal cavity [13,30–33]. In these procedures the distal portion of one of the horns of the bicornuate uterus is removed and cut into 2 to 5 mm squares and sutured to various positions within the peritoneal cavity (Fig. 2). Although all surgically transplanted uterine squares will implant and grow regardless of implantation site, Vernon and Wilson found that implantations adjacent to blood vessels (e.g., mesenteric arterial arcades) will grow larger than those in less vascular areas (e.g., ovarian fat pad) [13]. As with the monkey [23], implantation of uterine tissue in the rat does not require estrogen priming or collection of tissue during estrus [13,30–33].

Surgical procedures that are less invasive to the reproductive tract of the rat, unfortunately, have not been developed. The dissemination of isolated endometrial cells from uterine washings or scrapings from the uterine lumen have not been found to have the capacity to implant within the peritoneal cavity of the rat [13]. Therefore, surgical induction of endometriosis in the rat currently requires the removal of the distal portion of one uterine horn, thus leaving these rats with only a unilaterally intact reproductive tract.

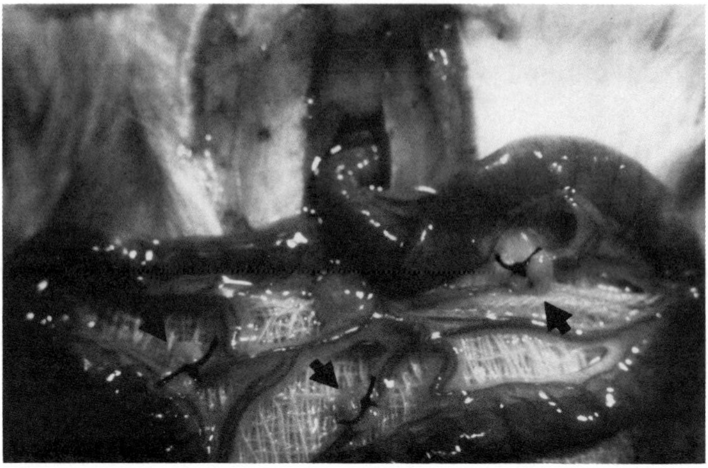

Fig. 2. Surgically exposed abdominal viscera of the rat showing (arrows) placement of autotransplanted uterine squares (Reprinted with permission from Fertil Steril 44:684, 1985).

In a novel approach for using the rodent as a model for endometriosis, Zamah and coworkers [34] injected human uterine and endometriotic implant endometrium into athymic mice. These immunologically suppressed mice have a congenital thymus aplasia [35] that leaves the animal with an impaired T-lymphocyte system and a deficiency in serum immunoglobulins [36]. The heterologous transplantation of uterine endometrial [34,37] and endometriotic implant tissue [34] from the human to athymic mice was found to implant, grow and respond to steroids.

Experimental Observations

The endometrium of the uterine squares autotransplanted to the peritoneal cavity of the rat (Fig. 2) grows in a fashion comparable to intact endometrium. These implants develop into highly vascular, tear-shaped cysts that contain clear, serous fluid (Fig. 3A) [13,30–33]. Uterine squares appear to grow exponentially for the first 2 months after transplantation, but are then maintained at a constant size for the next 10 months (Fig. 4) [13,30]. This restrained growth may be a result of entrapment of growing endometrium by a thin connective tissue sheath that covers the peritoneal surface of the implants. The connective tissue may have also limited the escape of endometrial secretions from the surface of the implant and thus may be responsible for the cystic nature of the implants.

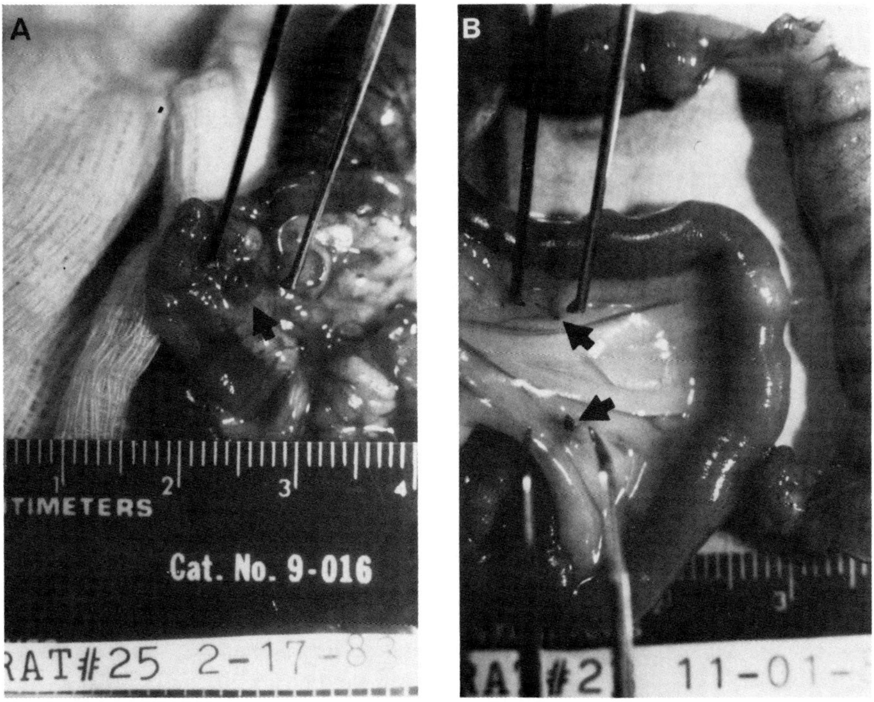

Fig. 3. Surgically exposed abdominal viscera of the rat showing (arrows) the appearance of endometriotic implants at approximately 40 days after autotransplantation in the nonpregnant rat (**A**) and pregnant rat (**B**). Note the total regression of implants in the pregnant animal (Reprinted with permission from Fertil Steril 44:684, 1985).

Histologically, the cystic implants contain stromal and endometrial epithelium that are similar to the endometrium. The inner lining of the cysts contains simple columnar epithelium with endometrial-like glands positioned at several positions along the interior of the cysts [13,30]. The lumen of the cysts contains free-floating endometrial cells and a large population of leukocytes [13,30]. Even though implants contained numerous leukocytes, at no time during a 10-month period of examination were implants observed to undergo histological necrosis [13]. As part of the pathophysiology of endometriosis, the body may be eliciting an autoimmune response against the endometriotic implant; however, the lack of cellular death would suggest that the immune response may not be against the endometrium, but instead against uterine secretions. Autoimmunity and other immunological dysfunctions [38]

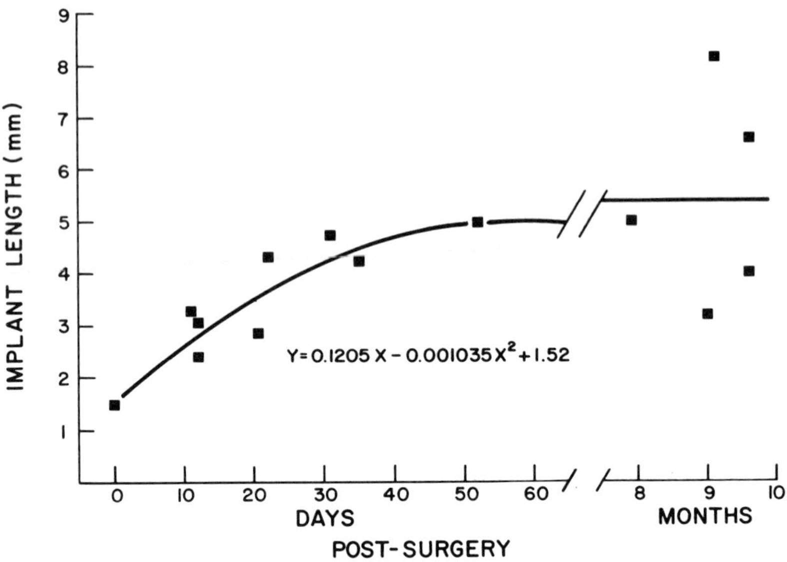

Fig. 4. The size of endometriotic implants at various times after autotransplantation. Each point represents the mean length of the four implants and the quadratic equation is the linear regression equation from day 0 to day 60 (Reprinted with permission from Fertil Steril 44:684, 1985).

have been suggested as playing a role in endometriosis, and the rat model may serve as a means to isolate the source of this response.

Prostaglandins have been suggested as one of the causative agents of the pain and infertility associated with endometriosis. Vernon and coworkers [13] measured the concentration of prostaglandin F (PGF) within implants of rats and found it to be similar to the amount measured in uteri (202 vs. 205 ng/mg tissue). These data are similar to human data, which indicate that implants contain and produce PGF [39] and also present evidence that the endometriotic implant of rats are biochemically active.

The endometriotic implant of the rat requires steroid stimulation for growth and development. Endometriotic implants will fail to grow in the adrenalectomized-ovariectomized rat but will show moderate growth in the ovariectomized (adrenal intact) rat due to the presence of adrenal progesterone [31]. If animals with fully developed implants are ovariectomized, the implants will undergo partial regression [32]. Thus steroids play an obligatory role in the development of the implant in the rat.

Implants appear to respond to steroids in a fashion similar to, but not the same as, uterine endometrium [31]. Implants will increase in size after 2 days of estrogen stimulation and this stimulation can be suppressed with progesterone. However, the response of the implant to steroids is not as vigorous as uterine endometrium. When cellular proliferation is measured with examination of a mitotic index, proliferation of the uterine endometrium is markedly stimulated by estrogen, whereas implants are only one-third as responsive. Furthermore, estrogen treatment will double the PGF content of the uterus but will be without effect on endometriotic implants [31]. Along these same lines, the impaired response of implants has also been noted in the human [40,41]. Enzyme-histochemical studies suggest that although enzymes, like alkaline phosphatase, are present in human implants, they are present in concentrations that are less than that of the uterus [40]. Additionally, the estrogen and progesterone receptor population is reduced in implants relative to the uterus [41]. The ectopic nature of the human and rat implant appears to reduce its biochemical and functional capacity. This reduced activity may be responsible, in part, for the infertility associated with endometriosis and needs to be investigated further in the human and animal models.

The efficacy of various drug treatments for endometriosis have been examined in the rat model. Long-term treatment of rats with endometriosis with levonorgestrel [32], estrogen, or progesterone [31] will maintain implants, but GnRH agonists will regress implant growth [32]. The regression of implants from GnRH agonists was transitory with implant regrowth occurring after drug withdrawal [32]. Danazol treatment for 2 weeks [31] or 3 weeks [32] moderately stimulated or had little effect on endometriotic implant growth. However, Dargenio and coworkers [42] elicited complete regression of implants after 4 weeks of superpharmacologic doses of danazol. From these data the most dramatic means of regressing ectopic endometrium was, therefore, through steroid withdrawal (i.e., GnRH agonists and ovariectomy).

As in the human, the presence of ectopic endometrium will impair the fertility of the rat [13]. Rats with endometriosis delivered 48% fewer pups and contained 28% fewer midgestational embryos than normal disease-free animals. Even though implants increased the number of pelvic adhesions, the reduced fecundity of rats was determined to be independent of adhesion formation and possibly involving anomalies with ovulation, fertilization, and embryo implantation [13]. The most striking result of this study was the suppressive influence of pregnancy upon implant growth. Autotransplanted implants more than doubled in size by 40 days after surgical implantation in the nonpregnant rat (Fig. 3A), whereas implants were not visible during this same period if rats became pregnant (Fig. 3B). During pregnancy, implants were histologically found to contain endometrial components that appeared to be viable, because implant growth resumed after parturition (Fig. 5).

Therefore, pregnancy, as with GnRH agonists, did not cure the disease but elicited temporary remission.

Summary

The rat has several attributes that make it appealing for use as a model for endometriosis. It is an inexpensive spontaneous ovulator whose reproductive cycle has been endocrinologically well defined. Surgical procedures are brief and can be performed without an operating room. A rat has 70 to 80 estrous cycles during the year, compared with 12 cycles in the monkey, and accordingly allows for the accumulation of more information in a shorter period of time. The rat, therefore, offers many experimental opportunities not available through human and nonhuman primate studies. The major deficiency of the rat as a model for endometriosis is the wide phylar gap between itself and the human. Because of this, care must be taken in interpreting the implication of rat studies relative to human endometriosis.

SURGICAL INDUCTION OF ENDOMETRIOSIS IN THE RABBIT

Reproductive Endocrinology

The rabbit (*Oryctolagus cuniculus*) is an induced ovulator and therefore does not have a discernible estrous cycle. Tertiary ovarian follicles are continuously developing (4–17 days) and regressing (1–2 days) in a fashion

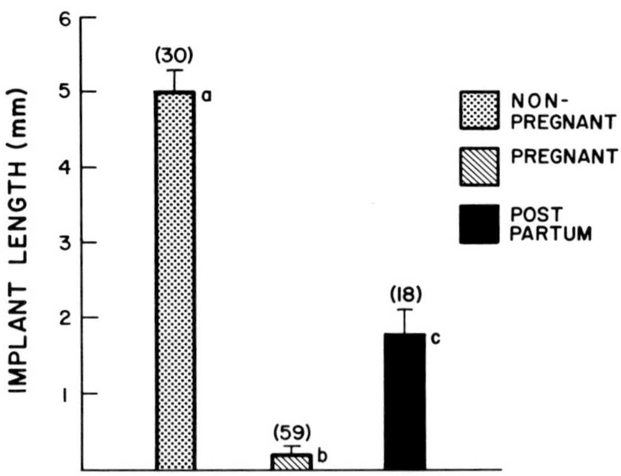

Fig. 5. Implant size in the nonpregnant, second trimester pregnant, and postpartum rat with surgically induced endometriosis. Each bar represents the mean $\pm$ standard error of the mean, and the numbered within parenthesis indicate sample size. Bars with different letter superscripts represent different means ($P < 0.05$; Reprinted with permission from Fertil Steril 44:684, 1985).

that produces a fairly constant number of follicles that are available for coitally induced ovulation. The vaginal lavage technique is not effective for the detection of "estrus" (i.e, peak estrogen); instead the appearance of the vulva, which under the influence of estrogen enlarges and becomes reddish to purple in color, could be monitored as an indication of peak follicular development. As an induced ovulator, the rabbit's reproductive pattern lacks a luteral phase and subsequently lacks the estrogen to progesterone pattern of the spontaneous ovulator.

Methodology

"Seeding" with fragments of endometrial tissue [10] or the suturing of endometrial squares to the peritoneal cavity [14,43–45] have both successfully led to implantation and growth of tissue. The distal portion of one of the uterine horns is usually removed as a source of endometrial tissue. The endometrium can be readily stripped from the myometrium and has been used as such by most current investigators. According to Weinstein and coworkers [43], estrogen pretreatment enhances the attachment of implants and several researchers have utilized this observation [14,46]. However, Hahn and coworkers [45] found that, in their hands, all autotransplanted endometrial tissue would implant without the additional need of steroid support. Likewise, Daniel and Williams-Boyce [47] utilized implants derived from untreated animals at "estrus" (i.e., swollen, red vulva) with complete success.

Experimental Observations

Sampson, in the 1920s, suggested that the etiology of endometriosis was through reverse regurgitation of menstrual components through the oviduct into the peritoneal cavity [8,9]. Realizing the value of an animal model for verification of this hypothesis, Jacobson, in 1922, surgically induced the disease by autotransplanting minced uterine tissue into the peritoneal cavity of the rabbit [10]. His 1-mm transplants of uterine tissue grew when implanted within the uterine wall, the ovary, and on the surface of the peritoneum. This validation of the ability of transplanted endometrial tissue to grow in vivo, and the concurrent verification by Cron of the viability of endometrial cells in human menstrual fluid [48] gave substantial, initial support to Sampson's reflux theory.

After transplantation, implants appear as vascularized hemorrhagic solid masses or multilocular cysts filled with a yellow serous fluid [10,14]. Hahn and coworkers [45] noted that implant growth was continuous for at least 15 weeks after implantation, with implant weight increasing from 10 mg at the time of implantation to 163 mg at week 15.

As also noted and discussed in the monkey and rat model, the endometriotic implants of the rabbit are responsive to hormones and drug therapies. Implants will regress after steroid withdrawal via oophorectomy [45] and were stimulated to grow by diethylstilbestrol diproprionate treatment [43]. Furthermore, implant weight and endometrial gland volume decreased in a dose-dependent fashion after 4 weeks of GnRH agonists or 8 weeks of danazol treatment [45].

The fertility of the rabbit is adversely affected by the presence of ectopic endometrial tissue. Schenken and Asch [14] noted a 50% reduction and Hahn and colleagues [44] a 53% reduction in the fertility rates of rabbits with induced endometriosis relative to sham controls. Both investigators found this reduced fertility to be independent of adhesion formation. Schenken and Asch [14] attributed the infertility to a defect in ovulation but could not exclude a postovulatory factor. Hahn and colleagues [44], on the other hand, did not observe any ovulatory dysfunction but suggested that the endometriosis impaired implantation of the embryos. An inverse correlation existed between the total amount of disease and the fertility rate of the rabbit ($R^2 = 0.708$). The number of ova implantations decreased as the total weight of endometriotic implants increased [44].

Summary

The rabbit has been used as a model for endometriosis by more researchers than any other species. The reason for this extensive utilization has been the ease of surgery (larger uterus than the rat), high success rate of tissue implantation, and low cost relative to the monkey. However, in addition to the phylar differences between the rabbit and human, a major criticism against the rabbit model is that it is not a spontaneous ovulator. Instead it is an induced ovulator and as such does not exhibit reproductive cycles or endocrine patterns that are similar to the human. However, as indicated by the many superb studies of the preceding section, the rabbit is still an excellent animal model that has already answered several difficult questions about endometriosis.

COMMENTS

Endometriosis remains an enigma among women's diseases. Although extreme care must be used when extrapolations are made between animal models and human conditions, the surgical induction of endometriosis in research animals serves as useful models for the study of those aspects of this disease that cannot be adequately examined directly in the human.

Several animal models have already been used to examine the etiology of endometriosis, the efficacy of drug treatments, the suppressive action of endometriosis upon fertility, the response of endometriosis to steroid modulation, and the role of prostaglandin production. Many other evasive questions about endometriosis beckon to be answered. Areas of research that need to be addressed include the pathophysio-mechanisms of endometriosis that are associated with ovulation, fertilization, embryo implantation, fecundity, adhesion formation, steroid cytosol receptors, prostaglandin production, luteal function, and autoimmunity. Finally, animal models offer several experimental avenues of corroborating clinical findings and for extending our knowledge to improved diagnosis and treatment of the pain and infertility associated with endometriosis in women.

REFERENCES

1. Jayle J: Le Solenome du ventre de la femme. Rev Franc de Gyn Obstet 21:285, 1926.
2. Cullen E: "Adenomyoma of the Uterus". Philadelphia and London: Saunders Book Co., 1908.
3. Meyer R: Ueber adenomatose Schleimhautwucherugen in der uterus und tubenwand und ihre pathologisch anatomische. Bedeutung Virch Arch 172:349, 1903.
4. McGoogan LS: Sterility and endometriosis. Arch Surg 59:437, 1949.
5. MacKenzie WF, Splitter GA, Valerio MG: Endometrosis in primates. Med Primatol 1:288, 1972.
6. Stilling D: Die entwicklung transplantierter Gewebsteile. Verh Dtsch Ges Pathol 6:122, 1903.
7. Nichols J: Implantation of tissue and its relation to cancer. J Med Res 13:187, 1904–05.
8. Sampson JA: Perforating hemorrhagic (chocolate) cysts of the ovary: their portions and especially their relation to pelvic adenomas of endometrial type. Arch Surg 3:245, 1921.
9. Sampson JA: Peritoneal endometriosis due to menstrual dissemination of endometrial tissue into peritoneal cavity. Am J Obstet Gynecol 14:422, 1927.
10. Jacobson VC: The autotransplantation of endometrial tissue in the rabbit. Arch Surg 5:281, 1922.
11. Jacobson VC: The intraperitoneal transplantation of endometrial tissue: an experimental study. Arch Pathol Lab Med 1:169, 1926.
12. Schenken RS, Asch RH, Williams RF, Hodgen GD: Etiology of infertility in monkeys with endometriosis: luteinized unruptured follicles, luteal phase defects, pelvic adhesions, and spontaneous abortions. Fertil Steril 41:122, 1984.
13. Vernon MW, Wilson EA: Studies on the surgical induction of endometriosis in the rat. Fertil Steril 44:684, 1985.
14. Schenken RS, Asch RH: Surgical induction of endometriosis in the rabbit: effect on fertility and concentration of peritoneal fluid prostaglandins. Fertil Steril 34:581, 1980.
15. Goodman AL, Hodgen GD: The ovarian triad of the primate menstrual cycle. Recent Prog Horm Res 39:1, 1983.
16. Valerio DA, Miller RL, Innes JRM, Courtney KD, Pallotta AJ, Guttmacher RM: "Macaca Mulatta, Management of a Laboratory Colony." New York, London: Academic Press, 1969.

17. Czaja JA, Robinson JA, Eiselle SG, Scheffler G, Goy RW: Relationship between sexual skin color of female Rhesus monkeys and midcycle plasma levels of oestradiol and progesterone. J Reprod Fertil 49:147, 1977.
18. Hartman CG: Studies in the reproduction of monkeys Macacus rhesus, with special reference to menstruation and pregnancy. Carnegie Inst. Wash., Contrib Embryol 23:1, 1932.
19. Fanton JW, Hubbard GB: Spontaneous endometriosis in a cynomolgus monkey (Macaca fascicularis). Lab Animal Sci 33:597, 1983.
20. MacKenzie WF: Animal model endometriosis in Rhesus monkeys. Am J Pathol 80:341, 1975.
21. TeLinde RW, Scott RB: Experimental endometriosis. Am J Obstet Gynecol 50:1147, 1950.
22. Scott RB, Wharton LR: The effects of estrone and progesterone on the growth of experimental endometriosis in Rhesus monkeys. Am J Obstet Gynecol 74:852 1957.
23. Dizerega GS, Barber DL, Hodgen GD: Endometriosis: role of ovarian steroids in initiation, maintenance, and suppression. Fertil Steril 33:649, 1980.
24. Ridley JH, Edwards KI: Experimental endometriosis in the human. Am J Obstet Gynecol 76:783, 1958.
25. Andrews MC, Andrews WC: Endometriosis. Am J Obstet Gynecol 78:776, 1959.
26. Hulme HB, Holmstrom EG: Stilbestrol treatment of dysmenorrhea. Obstet Gynecol 1:579, 1953.
27. Scott RB, Wharton LR: Effect of progesterone and norethindrone on experimental endometriosis in monkeys. Am J obstet Gynecol 84:867, 1962.
28. Scott RB, Wharton LR: The effect of excessive amounts of Diethystilbestrol on experimental endometriosis in monkeys. Am J Obstet Gynecol 69:773 1955.
29. American Fertility Society: Classification of endometriosis. Fertil Steril 32:633, 1979.
30. Vernon MW, Graves K, Jawad MJ, Wilson EA: The surgical induction of endometriosis in the rat. Thirtieth meeting of the society for Gynecologic Investigation, Washington, DC, 1983.
31. Vernon MW, Rush E, Wilson EA: Steroid modulation of endometriotic implants in rats with induced endometriosis. Thirty-first meeting of the society of Gynecologic Investigation, San Francisco, 1984.
32. Jones RC: The effect of a luteinizing hormone releasing (LRH) agonist (Wy-40,972), levonorgestrel, danazol and ovariectomy on experimental endometriosis in the rat. Acta Endocrinol 106:282, 1984.
33. Golan A, Winston RML, Dargenio R: Experimental endometriosis: a microsurgical animal model in rats. J Med Sci 20:1094, 1984.
34. Zamah NM, Dodson MG, Stephens LC, Buttram VC Jr, Besch PK, Kaufman RH: Transplantation of normal and ectopic human endometrial tissue into athymic nude mice. Am J Obstet Gynecol 149:591, 1984.
35. DeSousa MAB, Parrott DMV, Pantelouris EM: The lymphoid tissue in mice with congenital aplasia of the thymus. Clin Exp Immunol 4:637, 1969.
36. Sussdorf DH, McCann RL: Serum concentrations of four immunoglobulins in nonimmunized and immunized athymic "nude" mice. Immunochemistry 12:607, 1975.
37. Bergqvist A, Jeppsson S, Kullander S, Ljungberg O: Human endometrium transplanted into nude mice: histological effects of various steroid hormones. Am J Pathol 119:336, 1985.

38. Halme J, Becker S, Hammond MG, Raj MHJ, Raj S: Increased activation of pelvic macrophages in infertile women with mild endometriosis. Am J Obstet Gynecol 145:333, 1983.
39. Vernon MW, Beard JS, Graves K, Wilson E: Classification of endometriotic implants by morphologic appearance and capacity to synthesize prostaglandin F. Fertil Steril 46:801, 1986.
40. Parakash S, Ulfelder H, Cohen RB: Enzyme-histochemical observations on endometriosis. Am J Obstet Gynecol 91:990, 1965.
41. Janne O, Kauppila A, Kokko E, lantoo JT, Ronnnberg L, Vihko R: Estrogen and progestin receptors in endometriosis lesions: comparison with endometrial tissue. Am J Obstet Gynecol 141:562, 1981.
42. Dargenio R, Golan A, Winston RML: Experimental endometriosis and fertility: compared effects of an antigonadotropin (danazol) and an antiprostagladin (indomethacin). Acta Eur Fertil 15:257, 1984.
43. Weinstein BB, Weed JC, Collins CG, Lock FR, Schlosser JV: The effect of diethylstilbestrol diproprionate on endometrial transplants. Endocrinology 27:903, 1940.
44. Hahn DW, Carraher R, Foldesy R, McGuire JL: Studies on the mechanism of infertility associated with endometriosis and the effect of an LHRH agonist (Histrelin;ORF 17070) in an animal model for endometriosis. In Labrie F, Belanger A, Dupont A, (eds): "LHRH and its Analogues." Amsterdam: Elsevier Science Publishers, p. 203, 1984.
45. Hahn DW, Carraher RP, Foldesy RG, McGuire JL: Development of an animal model for quantitatively evaluating effects of drugs on endometriosis. Fertil Steril 44:410, 1985.
46. Keye WR, Matson GA, Dixon J: The use of the argon laser in the treatment of experimental endometriosis. Fertil Steril 39:26, 1983.
47. Daniel JC, Boyce-Williams PK: Surgical induction of endometriosis. In Daniels JC (ed): "Methods in Mammalian Reproduction." New York: Academic Press, p. 545, 1978.
48. Cron RL, Gey G: The viability of cast-off menstrual endometrium. Am J Obstet Gynecol 13:645, 1927.

Index